Be the Best You Can Be in Sport

The Daily Journal

'Journal Your Next 12 Weeks'

By Paul Kilgannon

Part of the Be the Best You Can Be In Sport Series

Copyright 2022 © Paul Kilgannon
All rights reserved.
Published by The Book Hub Publishing Group

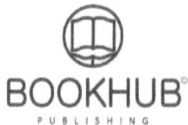

For further information re national & international distribution:
www.carvercoachingframework.com

ISBN: 978-1-7398725-9-5

All rights reserved. No part of this book may be used or reproduced in any manner whatsoever without the written permission of the publisher.
A catalogue record for this book is available from the British Library.

This publication is sold with the understanding that the Publisher/Author is not engaged in rendering health, legal services or other professional services. If legal advice, health or other expert assistance is required, the services of a competent, qualified professional person should be sought.

*Book Hub Publishing is committed to inclusion and diversity. We use paper sourced from sustainable forestry.

Name

Journal Start Date

Journal Number (If you don't know the answer… the answer is 1 ☺)

My hope and intention for this journal…

What am I looking to create and cultivate over the next 12 weeks?

Table of Contents

Introduction i

How to Use This Journal? iii

Your 'This is Me' Guide 3

This is Me 5

My Next Four Weeks 11

Tools to Drive Learning, Improvement and Performance in Sport 12

My Learning Tools 13

Goals & Intentions 17

My Goals – My Intentions 19

Tracking 21

My Tracker 22

My Next Four Weeks – Important Things 23

Week 1 24

Week 2 42

Week 3 60

Week 4 78

My Four-Week Review 96

My Next Four Weeks 99

My Learning Tools 100

My Goals – My Intentions 104

My Tracker 106

My Next Four Weeks – Important Things	107
Week 5	108
Week 6	126
Week 7	144
Week 8	162
My Four-Week Review	180
My Next Four Weeks	183
My Learning Tools	184
My Goals – My Intentions	188
My Tracker	190
My Next Four Weeks – Important Things	191
Week 9	192
Week 10	210
Week 11	228
Week 12	246
My Four-Week Review	264
My Quarterly Review	266
My New 'This is Me' Guide	270
This is Me	271
Reflections on 12 Weeks of Journaling	277
The End is Always the Beginning	279

Introduction

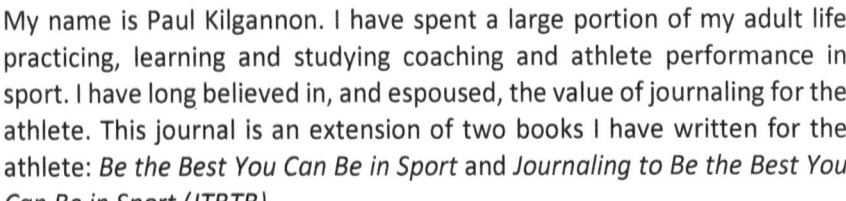

My name is Paul Kilgannon. I have spent a large portion of my adult life practicing, learning and studying coaching and athlete performance in sport. I have long believed in, and espoused, the value of journaling for the athlete. This journal is an extension of two books I have written for the athlete: *Be the Best You Can Be in Sport* and *Journaling to Be the Best You Can Be in Sport (JTBTB)*.

It is not necessary for you to have read *Be the Best You Can Be in Sport*, but it may be of interest to you. However, in order to maximise the potential of this journal, it is recommended that you have read and completed *JTBTB* prior to starting this journal. *JTBTB* is a precursor to this journal and is a deep dive into the art form of journaling for wellbeing and improved sporting performance. It challenges you to complete thirty days of demanding journaling practices and prompts. Throughout this journal I will consistently reference you back to insights, tools and techniques that are explained and explored in *JTBTB*. For those of you who do not complete *JTBTB* I have provided a series of useful videos in the *Resources* section of the *Blog* on my website- www.carvercoachingframework.com. You will find the QR code link to this on the next page.

This journal is a 12-week (quarterly) day-to-day journal that is designed to become your constant companion as you live your way through sport and life. Once you have completed one quarterly journal, you begin a new one. For it to be of continued value, journaling is something that must be consistently practiced. You must continue to self-invest. The mastery is in the process.

This journal is a system that will help you build good practices and habits as you go. Good systems and habits build the momentum required to be a self-managing athlete.

"You do not rise to the level of your goals. You fall to the level of your systems."

— James Clear, Atomic Habits

Simple habits and practices preformed consistently over time have a great impact. Sport (and life) is a 'learning competition' and a game of continual adjustment. This world is complex and uncertain. Circumstance and situation push and pull us in different directions on a daily basis. It is how we respond to this that determine our outcomes.

This journal is a tool designed to help you discern the huge volume of information the modern world challenges you to process on a daily basis.

"We are drowning in information, but starved for knowledge."

— John Naisbitt, Megatrends

This journal is designed to help you learn and develop as both a person and athlete. My hope is that it will lead you to a consistent state of growth and progress. My hope is that this journal is of service to you.

Be the best you can be,
Paul Kilgannon

This link will bring you to a series of useful videos that will help you with many of the tools and skills mentioned throughout this journal.

How to Use This Journal?

This journal is created as somewhat of a blank canvas for you in journaling. It cannot be too prescriptive or restrictive. It must merely act as a guide or framework for you. You can complete some, or all, of the challenges, prompts and practices included. It is your journal. How you use it is up to you.

Do what works for you...work it as you please... the important thing is that work is done.

I have broken this quarterly (12 weeks) journal into thirds (four-week blocks). The four-week blocks will act as a 28-day cycle within the quarter, making it easier for you to plan ahead, navigate different blocks of your year, measure progress and in general, manage the process of trying to be the best you can be.

As stated previously, in order to use this journal to its potential it is recommended you have completed JTBTB. That book details many of the journaling, planning and performance tools and techniques that will be referred to here.

As in *JTBTB*, this journal begins and ends with your 'This is Me' guide. This is a critical part of the journal as performance in sport both begins and ends with really knowing oneself and being clear on who you are, who you want to be and how you want to live, prepare and perform. Throughout the journal you will also be continually challenged to reflect on the content of this guide. JTBTB will have guided you through this process in great detail and given you an appreciation of its importance.

Your daily journaling will begin on a Sunday. My advice to you initially is to take a few days before this to:

1. Complete your 'This is Me' guide.
2. Set some clear goals or intentions for the next four weeks (the first third of this quarter.)
3. Develop tools that will help you: plan, measure, track, learn, reflect and so on.

4. Establish what you would like to track and measure over the next four weeks.

Wise men say only fools rush in.

I urge you to take the time required to complete this work before commencing this journal on a Sunday.

Throughout this journal, Sundays will be used to plan for the week ahead and bring clarity with regard to how you want to spend your time and live your days. Every Sunday you will find 8 journaling prompts, with each prompt assigned a number. The following 2 pages are blank allowing you to journal to the prompts of your choice; simply write the number of the prompt and journal your response. **I would urge you to complete three of the prompts at the very least and hope that you would complete more and perhaps all of them; this is important work.** To quote the writer Annie Dillard, *"How we spend our days is, of course, how we spend our lives."* Life is simply a collection of days.

"Every Sunday I'd write a plan for the week. I didn't want to waste any day. I'd plan days off. I was really strict in my preparation. I think that was a big part in my success and my drive."

— Dan Carter

On the Saturdays, you will be challenged to reflect on your learnings from the previous week and gain insights from these learnings. Similar to the Sundays, every Saturday you will find 14 journaling prompts, with each prompt assigned a number. The following 3 pages are blank allowing you to journal to the prompts of your choice; simply write the number of the prompt and journal your response. **Here, I would urge you to complete five of the prompts at the very least and hope that you would complete more; this is important work.** In sport your only sustainable competitive advantage is to learn faster and better than your opponents. In order to do so you must be a proactive learner.

"We do not learn from experience... we learn from reflecting on experience."

— John Dewey

These two days are critical for you, so high quality time is needed here. Both days will require you to spend twenty to thirty minutes on planning and reflection. Every fourth Saturday and Sunday, will require you to spend a little more time in reflection, contemplation and planning as you bring to end one four-week block and begin a new one.

It must be acknowledged that using Sunday as the beginning point of the week and Saturday as the end point of the week may not work for every athlete in every situation; for example, you have an important competition on a Sunday. Again, I ask you to use your discretion and intuition here and be flexible in situations like this. Also, this journal is designed to be used by the athlete at any time of their year: off- season, pre- season, or in-season. The hope is the four-week blocks will help with this and again, the advice is to use the journal as best works for you at any given time.

Embrace flexibility throughout this journal.

The weekdays will be used for simple morning and evening journaling exercises. Here you will find three journaling prompts at the top of each page, with each prompt assigned a number. The rest of the page is blank. **This gives you two options: you can journal to one, two or three of the prescribed prompts (simply write the number and your journal response) or journal freely as you please simply noting observations and thoughts about daily events, happenings, learnings, feelings etc.** (this journaling style can be referred to as *Stream of Conscious Journaling*.) The choice is yours and you can pick and choose how you proceed from one day to the next. Indeed, on certain days you may wish to use the journaling space provided in a more sports orientated manner in order to sharpen your focus prior to an important challenge. For example, you might like to use the space to set your points of focus or intentions prior to training or a game.

Each day includes a *Morning Wellbeing Check-In* and *Evening Wellbeing Markers* section. These are to be completed in the morning upon rising and in the evening as part of your journaling. It is a 5-star rating across four categories (morning and evening) which will give you a *Total Score*.

- Being measured in the morning are: Sleep (amount and quality), Energy Levels, Mood and Muscle Soreness. 1 star indicates *very poor* and 5 stars indicates *excellent*. In the case of Muscle Soreness, a 5-star rating would mean you have no muscle soreness and feel excellent in that category.

- Being measured in the evening are: Hydration (between 2 to 3 litres is great depending on activity levels), Nutrition (amount and quality), Daylight/Outside (time outside in daylight and nature each day…30 minutes is great) and Phone (the mindful, conscious, productive and healthy use of your phone). Again, 1 star indicates *very poor* and 5 stars indicates *excellent.*

I advise you to complete these on a consistent basis as they will give you great insight into your health and wellbeing over time.

Also, on most weekday mornings, you will be challenged to revert back to your 'This is Me' guide in one form or another. These exercises are used in order to really get to know and understand what is important to you as a person and athlete.

Within each four-week block there will be four different sets of daily prompts (one set per week for the four weeks). These four different sets of daily prompts will be repeated throughout each four-week block. Your weekday journaling will take approximately fifteen minutes of your day in total. If you feel like giving more time to it, then by all means go ahead. Again the message is simple:

Do what works for you…work it as you please… the important thing is that work is done.

You can almost always control how your day starts and ends, therefore setting routines for these times is relatively easier. Journaling in the morning sets the tone for the day and this is when its impact is strongest.

One of the challenges of journaling is actually consistently making time to do it and embed it as a habit. Here, you will have to push yourself and hold yourself accountable and responsible.

"The moment you take responsibility for everything in your life is the moment you can change anything in your life."

— Hal Elrod

To make the required time, you may need to set the clock ten minutes earlier than usual in the morning or spend ten minutes less on TV or screen time in the evening. I challenge you to look at journaling as 'special time' and this perspective will energise you. Your journaling time should be viewed as 'the best time' of your day.

> *"The important thing is to keep the important thing, the important thing."*
>
> — Albert Einstein

If you miss a day of journaling, don't worry, simply get back to it the following day; try not to miss twice in a row.

Consistency is king.

The Appendix of *JTBTB* provided you with tools that are generic in nature and may be of help to you. These tools are designed to provide basic and rudimental templates you may wish to modify or adapt. As noted in *JTBTB*, it will take a significant effort on your behalf to come up with your own set of personalised tools that will be of genuine value to you. However, if you wish to be the best you can be in sport, be assured that this will be time well spent. Again, I suggest you take the time to develop, or refine, some of these tools before beginning this journal on a Sunday and I have provided space for you to do this at the beginning of each four-week cycle (see pages 100 - 184). Understand and appreciate that you will improve and become more efficient in designing, developing and refining tools as you go.

Think progress and improvement rather than perfection.

This journal is full of prompts and challenges which only you can answer. It will give you the opportunity to build and nurture your personal and sporting identity and behaviours, which, in turn, will allow you to focus on who you are and who you are going to become. This journal will challenge you in many ways.

> *"Nothing worth having was ever achieved without effort."*
>
> — Theodore Roosevelt

Finally, in order to bring this journal to life and make it into something truly special, I suggest you personalise it any way you see fit: use colour, sketch and draw on it, highlight things of importance, perhaps write as neatly as you can, and from time to time reread and reflect on what you have written.

To end, I will again direct those who do not complete *JTBTB* to a series of useful videos in the *Resources* section of the *Blog* on my website www.carvercoachinframework.com. See the QR code provided on page ii.

Enjoy the journey!

24 Things to Always Remember...and One Thing to Never Forget

By Colin McCarty

Your presence is a present to the world.
You're unique and one of a kind.
Your life can be what you want it to be.
Take the days just one at a time.
Count your blessings, not your troubles.
You'll make it through whatever comes along.
Within you are so many answers.
Understand, have courage, be strong.
Don't put limits on yourself.
So many dreams are waiting to be realised.
Decisions are too important to leave to chance.
Reach for your peak, your goal, your prize.
Nothing wastes more energy than worrying.
The longer one carries a problem, the heavier it gets.
Don't take things too seriously.
Live a life of serenity, not a life of regrets.
Remember that a little love goes a long way…
Remember that a lot…goes forever.
Remember that friendship is a wise investment.
Life's treasures are people…together.
Realise that it's never too late.
Do ordinary things in an extraordinary way.
Have health and hope and happiness.
Take time to wish upon a star.
And don't ever forget…for even a day…
How very special you are.

Wise Men Say, Only Fools Rush In...

Before beginning your journaling adventure, please take a breath and ensure you have read the previous pages. They are full of instruction, information and insights that will prepare you for what is to come and allow you to get the most out of this journal.

Your 'This is Me' Guide

Your first challenge is to complete your 'Personal Manifesto' or 'This is Me' guide. This guide was a central part of *JTBTB* and it is important that you have completed it in detail in order to fully engage with what is to follow. It is advised that you return to pages 133-136 (or if not, pages 52-55) of *JTBTB* to review the work who have completed here to date and use this as your starting point. For those who do not complete *JTBTB* I again refer you to the *Resources* section of the *Blog* on my website www.carvercoachinframework.com. Here you will find a useful video to help you with your 'This is Me' guide (see the QR Code provided on page ii).

I urge you to go deep here and to be honest and open. This guide will be central to the process. The depth of attention this work was given in *JTBTB* is the main reason I recommend you complete *JTBTB* in advance of beginning this journal.

Once completed, the below guide should act as an *anchor* or *North Star* as you move forward over the next quarter. It is a snapshot of who you are, who you want to be and how you want to live inside of and outside of sport at this point in time. It should act as a go-to 'source' for you to come and seek direction on a daily basis.

> *"My success in the ring doesn't mean as much as my integrity... that's definitely the most important thing to me."*
>
> — Katie Taylor

Through your journaling and life experiences you will learn much that may lead you to change and refine this guide, making it more meaningful, unique and authentic to you. This guide will continue to change and evolve as a document, as you continue to change and evolve as a person and athlete. My advice to you is to swap any expectation you may have of perfection with an appreciation of refinement and progress.

"I am never going to arrive at who I am ... I can keep exploring... I'm on this amazing journey... I'll (always) be thinking about who I could be."

— Jonny Wilkinson

Life, and indeed sport, is about unpacking the most difficult question of "Who am I?"

"We have never arrived. We are in a constant state of becoming."

— *Bob Dylan*

This is Me

My name is _____

I am more than just a _____
(Sport you play)

I play _____

The areas of my life that are most important to me are:

_____
_____
_____
_____
_____

My *Values* are: (Please add a definition or standard of behaviour for each one.)

_____
_____
_____
_____
_____
_____
_____
_____
_____
_____
_____
_____
_____
_____

This is Me

My *Personal Mission Statement* is:

_____
_____
_____
_____
_____
_____
_____
_____

What sport means to me:

_____
_____
_____
_____
_____
_____
_____
_____

I want to be remembered by those I played sport with and against as someone who:

_____
_____
_____
_____
_____
_____
_____
_____

This is Me

My vision for myself as a teammate is:
_____
_____
_____
_____
_____
_____
_____

As an athlete, my current *weapons* are:
_____
_____
_____
_____

As an athlete, my current *work-ons* are:
_____
_____
_____
_____

To ensure I learn as I go in sport, I utilise the following tools and practices:
_____
_____
_____
_____
_____
_____
_____

This is Me

My truth or belief around application to collective and individual practice is: (i.e. how I believe one should best apply themselves to practice.)

_____
_____
_____
_____
_____
_____
_____

The activities and hobbies outside of sport that give me energy, bring me joy and add balance to my life are:

_____
_____
_____
_____
_____
_____
_____

With regard to how I spend my time and energy, I aim to be a person who:

_____
_____
_____
_____
_____
_____
_____
_____

This is Me

My personal definition of *Excellence* is:

_____
_____
_____
_____
_____

My personal definition of *Commitment* is:

_____
_____
_____
_____

My personal definition of *Success* is:

_____
_____
_____
_____
_____

Anything else you'd like to add:

_____
_____
_____

Signed: _____ **Date:** _____

My Next Four Weeks

Tools to Drive Learning, Improvement and Performance in Sport

In the appendix of *JTBTB* (see the QR Code provided on page ii), tools of a generic nature were provided to help you plan, measure, track, learn, reflect and so on. These were designed to provide basic and rudimental templates you may wish to modify or adapt. It will take a significant effort on your behalf to come up with your own set of personalised tools that will be of genuine value to you and indeed the help of professionals may well be required in this. If you wish to be the best you can be in sport, be assured that this will be time well spent.

"A good tool improves the way you work. A great tool improves the way you think."

—Jeff Duntemann

You don't necessarily need to develop all these tools at once, or to begin with. You can build your toolbox as you go. Again, consistency is king. The mastery is in sticking to a mindset of continuous improvement.

Useful tools may include:

- A Personal Improvement Plan for The 5 Pillars of the Athlete.
- A Sport Specific Personal Improvement Plan.
- A Personal Performance Analysis Tool.
- A Pre- Game Wheel of Preparation Tool.
- Affirmation Scripts.

My advice is that as you develop these tools you can create a master copy using the aid of a computer application such as Microsoft Word or Excel. Print them out and attach them to the blank pages which follow. Alternatively, you may wish to store them electronically or in a folder that you keep with your journal. The key is to simplify their storage and to have them at hand when you are journaling and reflecting.

At the beginning of each four-week block, space will be provided for tools. Some of these tools may remain the same from block to block, will others may be modified, changed or improved. Again the message is simple:

Learn and grow as you go.

My Learning Tools

My Learning Tools

My Learning Tools

My Learning Tools

Goals & Intentions

In your 'This is Me' guide you were asked to list the areas of your life that are most important to you. These likely included areas such as family, sport, study, work, friendship, hobbies etc. On pages 147-148 of *JTBTB* you were a given a *Simple Guide To Setting Goals* that you may find useful (see the QR Code provided on page ii).

I would like you to list at least one goal for each of the important areas of your life. Indeed, you may wish to set more than one for some areas; sport for example. You can set them for the next four weeks which would be more short-term goals, or twelve weeks which would be more medium-term goals. You can also acknowledge any long-term goals you may have which will no doubt motivate you as you go. Again, there is a good deal of flexibility and scope for you to do as you find best here; this is a blank canvass for you. Some goals may change from four-week block to four-week block (i.e. the short-term ones) while others may remain the same and move from block to block. If you are setting an 'outcome goal' you should set a 'process goal' to help get you there. Process goals can be tracked in your metric tracker which follows (again, reference the appendix of *JTBTB*- see QR Code provided earlier).

Give goalsetting a go and aim for improvement rather than perfection. Understand and appreciate that you will improve and become more effective and efficient with your goalsetting as you go. Consider who are the people in your life who will support you to achieve your goals. Also, think about what may be some of the barriers to you achieving your goals and how will you overcome them.

An alternative to goalsetting is the concept of intentions. For some, this is a simpler, almost warmer way of looking at things. It can be as simple as setting an intention for the areas of your life that are most important to you. These intentions act like a compass for you. They are like a mission statement for each area of your life. They can be short and sweet or more detailed in some areas, like sport for example. You may not always hit the mark but they act as a guide for you. An example of an intention in the area of academia and study could be…

"With regard to how I approach my studies I am a person who is organised, diligent, consistent and positive. I appreciate that although my studies can be challenging I am blessed to have been given the opportunity to learn and better myself. I embrace every opportunity I am given to learn. This mindset helps me maximise my academic abilities."

As with most things in this journal I am giving you an element of free reign here. Go and set your own goals or intentions in a way that works for you now, and as you follow the process, you will learn as you go and find what works best for you. The message is simple:

Learn and grow as you go.

My Goals – My Intentions

Signed: _____ Date: _____

My Goals – My Intentions

Signed: _____ Date: _____

Tracking

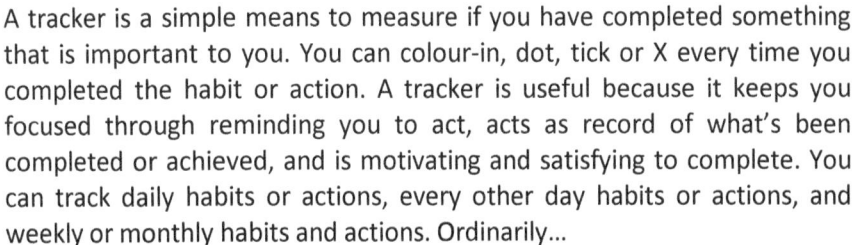

A tracker is a simple means to measure if you have completed something that is important to you. You can colour-in, dot, tick or X every time you completed the habit or action. A tracker is useful because it keeps you focused through reminding you to act, acts as record of what's been completed or achieved, and is motivating and satisfying to complete. You can track daily habits or actions, every other day habits or actions, and weekly or monthly habits and actions. Ordinarily…

What gets measured, gets done.

A personal metric is similar and describes a behaviour or action that is important to you with a quantifiable value. A daily/weekly/monthly hour count, is a personal metric that captures how much time you are spending in a particular area of your life. If something is important to you can track it with a number.

In the tracker provided you can simply write down an explainer, a SMART goal or the name of each habit or action you wish to track over the next four weeks and complete it as you go with the relevant value or symbol- be it either a number, an X or something similar.

I strongly advise that you track your use of your sporting 'tools' or any actions or behaviours associated with them. 'Habits create the future' and this is certainly the case in sport. You have developed these tools for a reason and tracking their use is certainly a good idea. I also advise you to track your adherence to the activities and hobbies outside of sport that give you energy, bring you joy and add balance and replenishment to your life.

It is also possible to track habits you are trying to break or areas/activities you are aiming to spend less time in. In truth, you can track anything you feel is important in any area of your life.

Finally, I will qualify the tracking and measuring of actions, habits and behaviours by acknowledging that…

Not everything that matters can be measured. Not everything that we can measure matters.

Again the message is simple:

Learn and grow as you go.

My Tracker

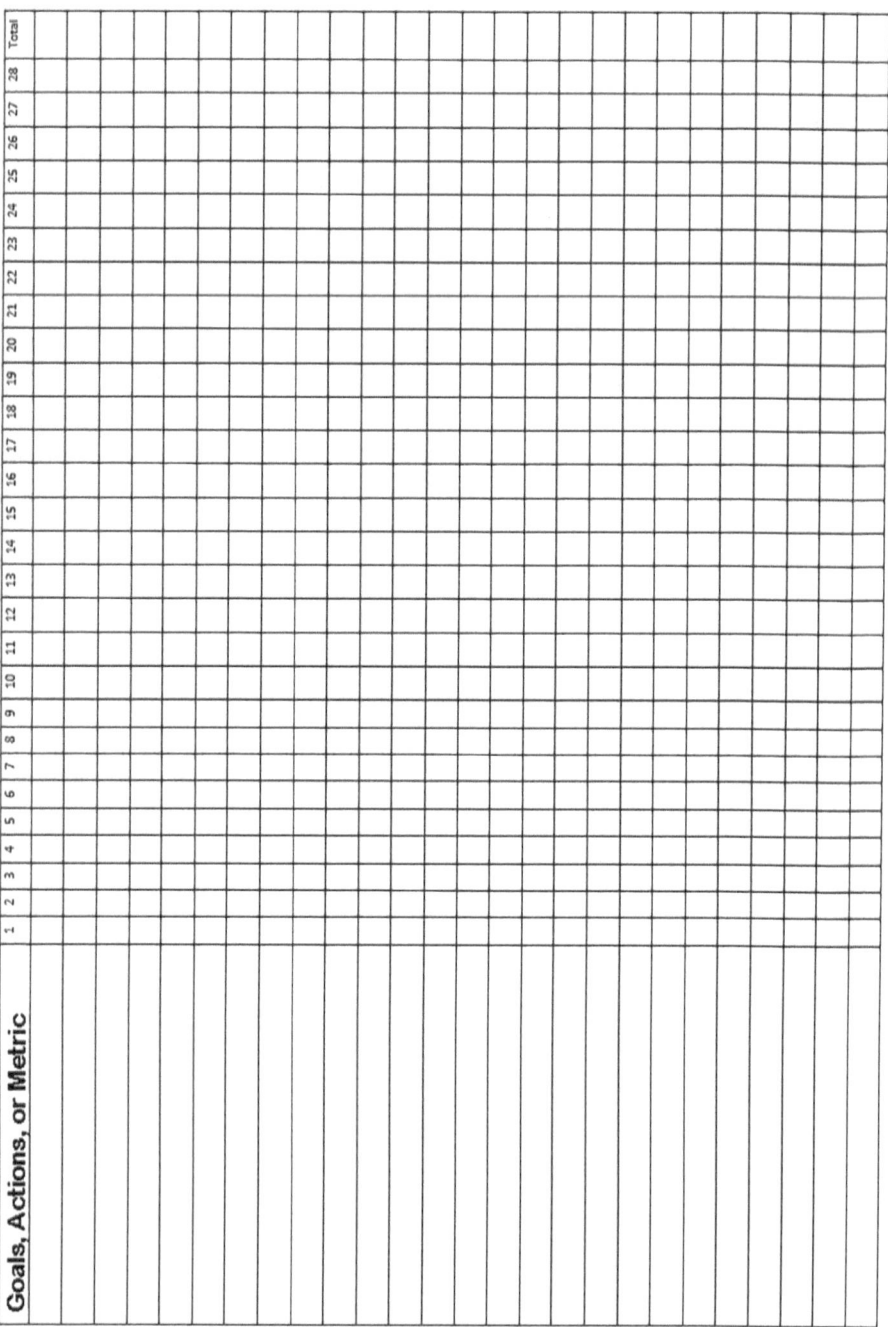

My Next Four Weeks – Important Things

(You can fill in the date in the small boxes provided in the top left-hand corner.)

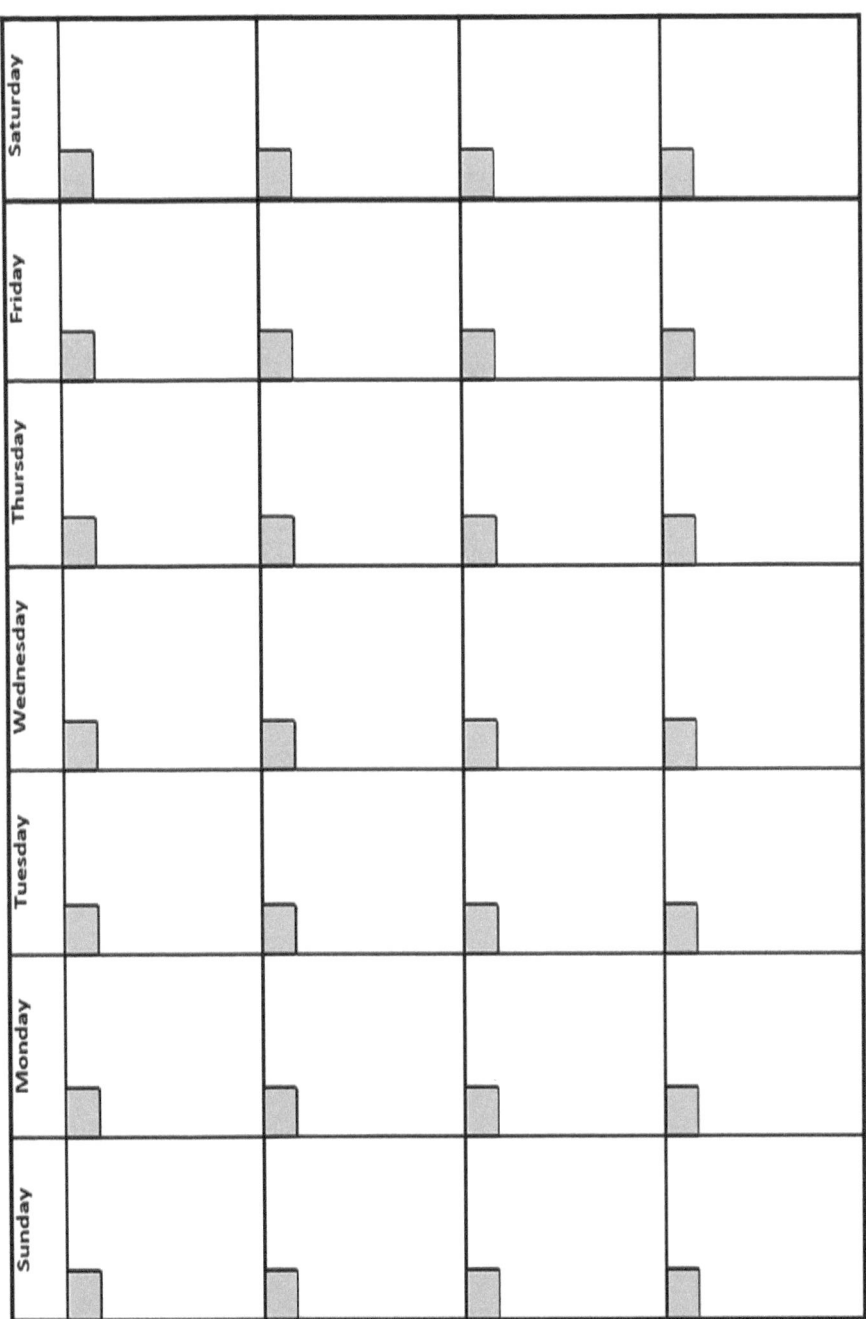

Sunday- Time to Plan for the Week Ahead

Date: _____

Your challenge is to complete three of these prompts at the very least; maybe more and perhaps even all of them. Simply write the number of the prompt and journal your response in the space provided. This is important work!

1) Describe in detail how you intend to live this week. Here you may wish to draw insights from your Values, your *Personal Mission Statement*, and your goals or intentions.
2) List at least one area of your life outside of sport that you would like to live with intention this week and explain the behaviours or actions required to do so.
3) Describe in detail at least one way you are going to improve as a teammate this week and explain how that will make you feel.
4) Describe in detail how you plan to improve as an athlete this week: what tools and practices are you going to utilise, what are your key *work-ons*, who or what can help you, etc.
5) What are the biggest sporting challenges that lay ahead of you this week? How to do want to 'show up' for these?
6) Full engagement is the acquired ability to give your full and best energy and effort to what you are doing at any given moment. Where is the one area you would like to be *fully engaged* this week and why is it important you do so?
7) In order to bring balance, recreation, regeneration and joy to your life this week what hobbies, interests or activities outside of sport do you need to make time for?
8) To help me make progress towards achieving my goals or living my intentions, this week I will…(List five actions.)

Important for the Week Ahead

Here you can use the blank spaces to schedule or craft your plan for the week ahead in whatever format you wish. Each day (and week) will be different, and plans may have to be flexible, but a solid plan for the week ahead is always a good idea. Spending some time to clarify your plans for the upcoming week will inform you how to best approach it. Feel free to jot down useful notes, intentions or ideas beside the event or activity.

"I don't care about three years ago. I don't care about two years ago. I don't care about last year. The only thing I care about is this week."

— Tom Brady

Monday	Tuesday	Wednesday
Thursday	Friday	Saturday

Monday- Date: _____

My Morning Wellbeing Check-In		Morning Prompts
Sleep ☆☆☆☆☆	Energy Levels ☆☆☆☆☆	1. What am I grateful for this morning? Explain in detail.
Mood ☆☆☆☆☆	Muscle Soreness ☆☆☆☆☆	2. How do I want to feel today and what am I willing to do to achieve this?
Total Wellbeing Score		3. I will smile when my head hits the pillow this evening if…

Morning Challenge- Return to page 5 and read your *Values* and their definitions three times.

My Evening Wellbeing Markers		Evening Prompts
Hydration ☆☆☆☆☆	Nutrition ☆☆☆☆☆	1. What did I do well today and why/how?
Daylight/Outside ☆☆☆☆☆	Phone ☆☆☆☆☆	2. What did I learn or relearn today?
Total Wellbeing Score		3. What is one thing I could have done better today and how?
Tick here when you have completed your habit/action/metric *tracker*.		

Tuesday- Date: _____			
My Morning Wellbeing Check-In			**Morning Prompts**
Sleep ☆☆☆☆☆	Energy Levels ☆☆☆☆☆		1. What am I grateful for this morning? Explain in detail.
Mood ☆☆☆☆☆	Muscle Soreness ☆☆☆☆☆		2. Who would I like to connect with today and why?
Total Wellbeing Score			3. What can I do in order to inject more fun into the day ahead?

Morning Challenge- Return to page 5 and read your *Values* and their definitions three times.

My Evening Wellbeing Markers		Evening Prompts
Hydration ☆☆☆☆☆	Nutrition ☆☆☆☆☆	1. What were the three best things about today?
Daylight/Outside ☆☆☆☆☆	Phone ☆☆☆☆☆	2. Who did I help today, how did I help them and how did it make me feel? Who could I have helped more?
Total Wellbeing Score		3. Something I am procrastinating over is... What action should I take?
Tick here when you have completed your habit/action/metric *tracker*.		

Wednesday- Date: _____

My Morning Wellbeing Check-In		Morning Prompts
Sleep ☆☆☆☆☆	Energy Levels ☆☆☆☆☆	1. What am I grateful for this morning? Explain in detail.
Mood ☆☆☆☆☆	Muscle Soreness ☆☆☆☆☆	2. Write about a positive experience from yesterday: what was it, why did it come about and how did it make you feel?
Total Wellbeing Score		3. I feel good when I start my day with….

_____
_____
_____
_____
_____
_____
_____
_____
_____
_____

Morning Challenge- Rewrite your *Values* and their definitions from memory and then return to page 5 to check for accuracy. Give it your best shot. Don't expect it to be perfect. It doesn't need to be.

_____
_____
_____
_____
_____
_____
_____
_____

My Evening Wellbeing Markers		Evening Journaling
Hydration ☆☆☆☆☆	Nutrition ☆☆☆☆☆	This is a *Stream of Consciousness Journaling* type of challenge. Simply write down all that comes to your mind below. There is no required outcome here, only to let whatever needs to come out... out. Write for ten minutes and use the blank pages provided at the back if necessary. Just... write!
Daylight/Outside ☆☆☆☆☆	Phone ☆☆☆☆☆	
Total Wellbeing Score		
Tick here when you have completed your habit/action/metric *tracker*.		

Thursday- Date: _____			
My Morning Wellbeing Check-In			**Morning Prompts**
Sleep ☆☆☆☆☆	Energy Levels ☆☆☆☆☆		1. What am I grateful for this morning? Explain in detail.
Mood ☆☆☆☆☆	Muscle Soreness ☆☆☆☆☆		2. What precisely is adding energy to my life right now?
Total Wellbeing Score			3. What is one thing I can do today to bring more happiness into my day?

Morning Challenge- Read your *Personal Mission Statement* from page 6 three times.

My Evening Wellbeing Markers		Evening Prompts
Hydration ☆☆☆☆☆	Nutrition ☆☆☆☆☆	1. Write about the highlight of your day; think- what, why, when, where, who and how.
Daylight/Outside ☆☆☆☆☆	Phone ☆☆☆☆☆	2. What did I learn or relearn today?
Total Wellbeing Score		3. How did I grow as an athlete and person today?
Tick here when you have completed your habit/action/metric *tracker*.		

Friday- Date: _____

My Morning Wellbeing Check-In		Morning Prompts
Sleep ☆☆☆☆☆	Energy Levels ☆☆☆☆☆	1. What am I grateful for this morning? Explain in detail.
Mood ☆☆☆☆☆	Muscle Soreness ☆☆☆☆☆	2. As I look towards the day ahead write down: two things I can control, two things I can influence and two things I can't control.
Total Wellbeing Score		3 What three things are most important for me today and how can I tend to these?

Morning Challenge- Rewrite your *Personal Mission Statement* from memory and then return to page 6 to check for accuracy. Give it your best shot. Don't expect it to be perfect. It doesn't need to be.

My Evening Wellbeing Markers		Evening Prompts
Hydration ☆☆☆☆☆	Nutrition ☆☆☆☆☆	1. What is currently bringing the most joy to my life and why?
Daylight/Outside ☆☆☆☆☆	Phone ☆☆☆☆☆	2. My greatest learning resources as an athlete are… (think: who, what, where, how).
Total Wellbeing Score		3. I live true to my values when I…
Tick here when you have completed your habit/action/metric *tracker*.		

Saturday- Date: _____
Time to Reflect and Summarise My Learnings

My Weekly Wellbeing Check-In Averages				
Sleep ☆☆☆☆☆	Energy Levels ☆☆☆☆☆	Hydration ☆☆☆☆☆	Nutrition ☆☆☆☆☆
Mood ☆☆☆☆☆	Muscle Soreness ☆☆☆☆☆	Daylight/Outside ☆☆☆☆☆	Phone ☆☆☆☆☆
My Average Wellness Score			
Out of 5, rate your consistency in using your habit/action/metric *tracker*			

Based on these scores, I need to:

Start _____

Stop _____

Continue _____

Your challenge is to complete five of these prompts at the very least; maybe more and perhaps even all of them. Simply write the number of the prompt and journal your response in the space provided. This is important work!

1) Note one example of how you lived according to your values/personal mission statement this week and explain how this made you feel.
2) Describe one way your values/personal mission statement were challenged or compromised this week and explain what you learned from this experience.
3) List two things that went well this week inside or outside of sport and offer reasons as to why.
4) What were your two most important learnings or relearnings this week (one inside sport and one outside of sport) and explain how you plan to bring these forward to better yourself?
5) What did you come across this week that you were interested in or were curious about, and would like to look into at a deeper level? How or where can you learn more about this?
6) Think of an example from the past week where you were *fully engaged*. Explain in detail how it felt to be *fully engaged*.
7) What relationships did I improve this week and how?
8) Who helped you this week and how?
9) I was a good teammate this week because…
10) I improved as an athlete this week by…
11) One great moment from the week I want to remember is…
12) My top three accomplishments from the week were:
13) Write a note on the progress you have made this week with regard to achieving your goals.
14) My key takeaways from this week are:

Sunday- Time to Plan for the Week Ahead

Date: _____

Your challenge is to complete three of these prompts at the very least; maybe more and perhaps even all of them. Simply write the number of the prompt and journal your response in the space provided. This is important work!

1) Describe in detail how you intend to live this week. Here you may wish to draw insights from your Values, your *Personal Mission Statement*, and your goals or intentions.
2) List at least one area of your life outside of sport that you would like to live with intention this week and explain the behaviours or actions required to do so.
3) Describe in detail at least one way you are going to improve as a teammate this week and explain how that will make you feel.
4) Describe in detail how you plan to improve as an athlete this week: what tools and practices are you going to utilise, what are your key *work-ons*, who or what can help you, etc.
5) What are the biggest sporting challenges that lay ahead of you this week? How to do want to 'show up' for these?
6) Full engagement is the acquired ability to give your full and best energy and effort to what you are doing at any given moment. Where is the one area you would like to be *fully engaged* this week and why is it important you do so?
7) In order to bring balance, recreation, regeneration and joy to your life this week what hobbies, interests or activities outside of sport do you need to make time for?
8) To help me make progress towards achieving my goals or living my intentions, this week I will…(List five actions.)

Important for the Week Ahead

Here you can use the blank spaces to schedule or craft your plan for the week ahead in whatever format you wish.

Monday	Tuesday	Wednesday

Thursday	Friday	Saturday

Monday- Date: _____	
My Morning Wellbeing Check-In	**Morning Prompts**
Sleep ☆☆☆☆☆ / Energy Levels ☆☆☆☆☆	1. List three things that are good about today.
Mood ☆☆☆☆☆ / Muscle Soreness ☆☆☆☆☆	2. Write the names of three people you interact with daily. Note at least one positive thing about each of them.
Total Wellbeing Score	3. How can I be kind to myself today?

Morning Challenge- Return to page 6 and read your explanation of, or answer to, 'What Sport Means to Me' three times.

My Evening Wellbeing Markers		Evening Prompts
Hydration ☆☆☆☆☆	Nutrition ☆☆☆☆☆	1. What is currently bringing satisfaction into my life?
Daylight/Outside ☆☆☆☆☆	Phone ☆☆☆☆☆	2. Where in my life am I currently making excuses? How can I improve this?
Total Wellbeing Score		3. I feel good when I end my day with...
Tick here when you have completed your habit/action/metric *tracker*.		

Tuesday- Date: _____

My Morning Wellbeing Check-In		Morning Prompts
Sleep ☆☆☆☆☆	Energy Levels ☆☆☆☆☆	1. List three things that are good about today.
Mood ☆☆☆☆☆	Muscle Soreness ☆☆☆☆☆	2. Who am I when I am at my very best (physically, mentally, spiritually, etc.)? Write between six to ten words that you believe are representative of you when you're most proud of yourself, regardless of circumstance or situation.
Total Wellbeing Score		3. Why is it important to be my authentic self?

Morning Challenge- Rewrite 'What Sport Means to Me' from memory and then return to page 6 to check for accuracy. Give it your best shot. Don't expect it to be perfect. It doesn't need to be.

My Evening Wellbeing Markers		Evening Prompts
Hydration ☆☆☆☆☆	Nutrition ☆☆☆☆☆	1. Three ways I was true to my *Values* today:
Daylight/Outside ☆☆☆☆☆	Phone ☆☆☆☆☆	2. List and explain at least two ways you feel like you are influencing others in a positive way.
Total Wellbeing Score		3. I am proud of myself today because…
Tick here when you have completed your habit/action/metric *tracker*.		

Wednesday- Date: _____			
My Morning Wellbeing Check-In			**Morning Prompts**
Sleep ☆☆☆☆☆	Energy Levels ☆☆☆☆☆		1. List three things that are good about today.
Mood ☆☆☆☆☆	Muscle Soreness ☆☆☆☆☆		2. What three things can I do today that will make me feel it was a great day when I reflect before I go to sleep?
Total Wellbeing Score			3. What is my most important 'Value' and why?

Morning Challenge- Return to page 7 and read your explanation for, or answer to, 'My Vision for Myself as a Teammate' three times.

My Evening Wellbeing Markers		Evening Journaling
Hydration ☆☆☆☆☆	Nutrition ☆☆☆☆☆	This is a *Stream of Consciousness Journaling* type of challenge. Simply write down all that comes to your mind below. There is no required outcome here, only to let whatever needs to come out... out. Write for ten minutes and use the blank pages provided at the back if necessary. Just... write!
Daylight/Outside ☆☆☆☆☆	Phone ☆☆☆☆☆	
Total Wellbeing Score		
Tick here when you have completed your habit/action/metric *tracker*.		

Thursday- Date: _____			
My Morning Wellbeing Check-In			**Morning Prompts**
Sleep ☆☆☆☆☆	Energy Levels ☆☆☆☆☆		1. List three things that are good about today.
Mood ☆☆☆☆☆	Muscle Soreness ☆☆☆☆☆		2. Write up a rough plan for the day ahead. Include the major events in your day and note how you wish to turn up and present yourself in each of these situations.
Total Wellbeing Score			3. Today I will…

Morning Challenge- Rewrite your 'My Vision for Myself as a Teammate' from memory and then return to page 7 to check for accuracy. Give it your best shot. Don't expect it to be perfect. It doesn't need to be.

My Evening Wellbeing Markers		Evening Prompts
Hydration ☆☆☆☆☆	Nutrition ☆☆☆☆☆	1. List three things that were good about today.
Daylight/Outside ☆☆☆☆☆	Phone ☆☆☆☆☆	2. Describe your biggest learning or relearning from today.
Total Wellbeing Score		3. Who helped me today and how did they help me?
Tick here when you have completed your habit/action/metric *tracker*.		

Friday- Date: _____		
My Morning Wellbeing Check-In		**Morning Prompts**
Sleep ☆☆☆☆☆	Energy Levels ☆☆☆☆☆	1. List three things that are good about today.
Mood ☆☆☆☆☆	Muscle Soreness ☆☆☆☆☆	2. How/Where/To whom do I want to show kindness today?
Total Wellbeing Score		3 What three things are most important to me for the day ahead?

My Evening Wellbeing Markers		Evening Prompts
Hydration ☆☆☆☆☆	Nutrition ☆☆☆☆☆	1. What did I do well today and why/how?
Daylight/Outside ☆☆☆☆☆	Phone ☆☆☆☆☆	2. Return to this morning's journal prompt where you were asked to list three things you felt were most important for you for the day ahead. Did you tend to these things in a satisfactory manner? If the answer is Yes: explain how this makes you feel. If the answer is No: explain your strongest reason for not doing it.
Total Wellbeing Score		3. What are the habits, behaviours or distractions that pull me away from being present or in the moment?
Tick here when you have completed your habit/action/metric *tracker*.		

Saturday- Date: _____
Time to Reflect and Summarise My Learnings

My Weekly Wellbeing Check-In Averages			
Sleep ☆☆☆☆☆	Energy Levels ☆☆☆☆☆	Hydration ☆☆☆☆☆	Nutrition ☆☆☆☆☆
Mood ☆☆☆☆☆	Muscle Soreness ☆☆☆☆☆	Daylight/Outside ☆☆☆☆☆	Phone ☆☆☆☆☆
My Average Wellness Score			
Out of 5, rate your consistency in using your habit/action/metric tracker			

Based on these scores, I need to:

Start _____

Stop _____

Continue _____

Your challenge is to complete five of these prompts at the very least; maybe more and perhaps even all of them. Simply write the number of the prompt and journal your response in the space provided. This is important work!

1) Note one example of how you lived according to your values/personal mission statement this week and explain how this made you feel.
2) Describe one way your values/personal mission statement were challenged or compromised this week and explain what you learned from this experience.
3) List two things that went well this week inside or outside of sport and offer reasons as to why.
4) What were your two most important learnings or relearnings this week (one inside sport and one outside of sport) and explain how you plan to bring these forward to better yourself?
5) What did you come across this week that you were interested in or were curious about, and would like to look into at a deeper level? How or where can you learn more about this?
6) Think of an example from the past week where you were *fully engaged*. Explain in detail how it felt to be *fully engaged*.
7) What relationships did I improve this week and how?
8) Who helped you this week and how?
9) I was a good teammate this week because...
10) I improved as an athlete this week by...
11) One great moment from the week I want to remember is...
12) My top three accomplishments from the week were:
13) Write a note on the progress you have made this week with regard to achieving your goals.
14) My key takeaways from this week are:

Sunday- Time to Plan for the Week Ahead

Date: _____

Your challenge is to complete three of these prompts at the very least; maybe more and perhaps even all of them. Simply write the number of the prompt and journal your response in the space provided. This is important work!

1) Describe in detail how you intend to live this week. Here you may wish to draw insights from your Values, your *Personal Mission Statement*, and your goals or intentions.
2) List at least one area of your life outside of sport that you would like to live with intention this week and explain the behaviours or actions required to do so.
3) Describe in detail at least one way you are going to improve as a teammate this week and explain how that will make you feel.
4) Describe in detail how you plan to improve as an athlete this week: what tools and practices are you going to utilise, what are your key *work-ons*, who or what can help you, etc.
5) What are the biggest sporting challenges that lay ahead of you this week? How to do want to 'show up' for these?
6) Full engagement is the acquired ability to give your full and best energy and effort to what you are doing at any given moment. Where is the one area you would like to be *fully engaged* this week and why is it important you do so?
7) In order to bring balance, recreation, regeneration and joy to your life this week what hobbies, interests or activities outside of sport do you need to make time for?
8) To help me make progress towards achieving my goals or living my intentions, this week I will...(List five actions.)

....
....
....
....
....
....
....
....
....
....
....
....

Important for the Week Ahead

Here you can use the blank spaces to schedule or craft your plan for the week ahead in whatever format you wish.

Monday	Tuesday	Wednesday

Thursday	Friday	Saturday

Monday- Date: _____		
My Morning Wellbeing Check-In		**Morning Prompts**
Sleep ☆☆☆☆☆	Energy Levels ☆☆☆☆☆	1. Complete this sentence three times: I am grateful for … because…
Mood ☆☆☆☆☆	Muscle Soreness ☆☆☆☆☆	2. Name one area you would like to be *fully engaged* today and explain why. We will refer to it this evening as your *fully engaged target area*.
Total Wellbeing Score		3. Write down some core principles for the day- What principles do I want to live by today?

_____
_____
_____
_____
_____
_____
_____
_____
_____
_____
_____
_____
_____
_____
_____
_____
_____
_____
_____
_____

Morning Challenge- Return to page 8 and read your explanation of, or answer to, 'My truth or belief around application to collective and individual practice' three times.

My Evening Wellbeing Markers		Evening Prompts
Hydration ☆☆☆☆☆	Nutrition ☆☆☆☆☆	1. How did your *fully engaged target area* from this morning play out for you? What lessons did you learn?
Daylight/Outside ☆☆☆☆☆	Phone ☆☆☆☆☆	2. Where have I been doing well of late? In what areas have I been growing?
Total Wellbeing Score		3. What am I currently finding inspiring?
Tick here when you have completed your habit/action/metric *tracker*.		

Tuesday- Date: _____

My Morning Wellbeing Check-In		Morning Prompts
Sleep ☆☆☆☆☆	Energy Levels ☆☆☆☆☆	1. Complete this sentence three times: I am grateful for ... because...
Mood ☆☆☆☆☆	Muscle Soreness ☆☆☆☆☆	2. Describe how you can behave and prepare like a champion today.
Total Wellbeing Score		3. Finish the following- I am... I can... I will...

Morning Challenge- Rewrite your 'My truth or belief around application to collective and individual practice' from memory and then return to page 8 to check for accuracy. Give it your best shot. Don't expect it to be perfect. It doesn't need to be.

My Evening Wellbeing Markers		Evening Prompts
Hydration ☆☆☆☆☆	Nutrition ☆☆☆☆☆	1. Champions consistently make good choices. Make a list of 'champion choices'.
Daylight/Outside ☆☆☆☆☆	Phone ☆☆☆☆☆	2. What did I learn or relearn today?
Total Wellbeing Score		3. Write about an area in your life where you feel stuck right now and how you can begin to make progress here.
Tick here when you have completed your habit/action/metric *tracker*.		

Wednesday- Date: _____			
My Morning Wellbeing Check-In		**Morning Prompts**	
Sleep ☆☆☆☆☆	Energy Levels ☆☆☆☆☆	1. Complete this sentence three times: I am grateful for ... because...	
Mood ☆☆☆☆☆	Muscle Soreness ☆☆☆☆☆	2. How can I have a positive impact on others today?	
Total Wellbeing Score		3. Today I will nourish my body and mind by...	

Morning Challenge- Return to page 9 and read your personal definition of *Excellence* three times.

My Evening Wellbeing Markers		Evening Journaling
Hydration ☆☆☆☆	Nutrition ☆☆☆☆☆	This is a *Stream of Consciousness Journaling* type of challenge. Simply write down all that comes to your mind below. There is no required outcome here, only to let whatever needs to come out... out. Write for ten minutes and use the blank pages provided at the back if necessary. Just... write!
Daylight/Outside ☆☆☆☆☆	Phone ☆☆☆☆☆	
Total Wellbeing Score		
Tick here when you have completed your habit/action/metric *tracker*.		

Thursday- Date:		
My Morning Wellbeing Check-In		**Morning Prompts**
Sleep ☆☆☆☆☆	Energy Levels ☆☆☆☆☆	1. Complete this sentence three times: I am grateful for ... because...
Mood ☆☆☆☆☆	Muscle Soreness ☆☆☆☆☆	2. Write for five minutes... 'I feel happiest when...' let it flow.
Total Wellbeing Score		3. How do I plan to grow as an athlete and person today?

Morning Challenge- Rewrite your personal definition of *Excellence* from memory and then return to page 9 to check for accuracy. Give it your best shot. Don't expect it to be perfect. It doesn't need to be.

My Evening Wellbeing Markers		Evening Prompts
Hydration ☆☆☆☆☆	Nutrition ☆☆☆☆☆	1. Much of sport involves dealing with discomfort, challenge and pressure. Write out a clear vision of how you want to show up in times of discomfort, challenge, and pressure. Take your time here; go deep, bring clarity.
Daylight/Outside ☆☆☆☆☆	Phone ☆☆☆☆☆	2. Where am I making real progress and why?
Total Wellbeing Score		3. I can add more depth to my life by…
Tick here when you have completed your habit/action/metric *tracker*.		

Friday- Date: _____

My Morning Wellbeing Check-In		Morning Prompts
Sleep ☆☆☆☆☆	Energy Levels ☆☆☆☆☆	1. Complete this sentence three times: I am grateful for ... because...
Mood ☆☆☆☆☆	Muscle Soreness ☆☆☆☆☆	2. Explain how you can bring your values into your interactions and experiences today.
Total Wellbeing Score		3. I find meaning and purpose in...

My Evening Wellbeing Markers		Evening Prompts
Hydration ☆☆☆☆☆	Nutrition ☆☆☆☆☆	1. What do I need to do more of and why?
Daylight/Outside ☆☆☆☆☆	Phone ☆☆☆☆☆	2. What do I need to do less of and why?
Total Wellbeing Score		3. What do I need to keep doing and why?
Tick here when you have completed your habit/action/metric *tracker*.		

Saturday- Date: _____
Time to Reflect and Summarise My Learnings

My Weekly Wellbeing Check-In Averages			
Sleep ☆☆☆☆☆	Energy Levels ☆☆☆☆☆	Hydration ☆☆☆☆☆	Nutrition ☆☆☆☆☆
Mood ☆☆☆☆☆	Muscle Soreness ☆☆☆☆☆	Daylight/Outside ☆☆☆☆☆	Phone ☆☆☆☆☆
My Average Wellness Score			
Out of 5, rate your consistency in using your habit/action/metric tracker			

Based on these scores, I need to:

Start _____

Stop _____

Continue _____

Your challenge is to complete five of these prompts at the very least; maybe more and perhaps even all of them. Simply write the number of the prompt and journal your response in the space provided. This is important work!

1) Note one example of how you lived according to your values/personal mission statement this week and explain how this made you feel.
2) Describe one way your values/personal mission statement were challenged or compromised this week and explain what you learned from this experience.
3) List two things that went well this week inside or outside of sport and offer reasons as to why.
4) What were your two most important learnings or relearnings this week (one inside sport and one outside of sport) and explain how you plan to bring these forward to better yourself?
5) What did you come across this week that you were interested in or were curious about, and would like to look into at a deeper level? How or where can you learn more about this?
6) Think of an example from the past week where you were *fully engaged*. Explain in detail how it felt to be *fully engaged*.
7) What relationships did I improve this week and how?
8) Who helped you this week and how?
9) I was a good teammate this week because…
10) I improved as an athlete this week by…
11) One great moment from the week I want to remember is…
12) My top three accomplishments from the week were:
13) Write a note on the progress you have made this week with regard to achieving your goals.
14) My key takeaways from this week are:

Sunday- Time to Plan for the Week Ahead

Date: _____

Your challenge is to complete three of these prompts at the very least; maybe more and perhaps even all of them. Simply write the number of the prompt and journal your response in the space provided. This is important work!

1) Describe in detail how you intend to live this week. Here you may wish to draw insights from your Values, your *Personal Mission Statement*, and your goals or intentions.
2) List at least one area of your life outside of sport that you would like to live with intention this week and explain the behaviours or actions required to do so.
3) Describe in detail at least one way you are going to improve as a teammate this week and explain how that will make you feel.
4) Describe in detail how you plan to improve as an athlete this week: what tools and practices are you going to utilise, what are your key *work-ons*, who or what can help you, etc.
5) What are the biggest sporting challenges that lay ahead of you this week? How to do want to 'show up' for these?
6) Full engagement is the acquired ability to give your full and best energy and effort to what you are doing at any given moment. Where is the one area you would like to be *fully engaged* this week and why is it important you do so?
7) In order to bring balance, recreation, regeneration and joy to your life this week what hobbies, interests or activities outside of sport do you need to make time for?
8) To help me make progress towards achieving my goals or living my intentions, this week I will…(List five actions.)

Important for the Week Ahead

Here you can use the blank spaces to schedule or craft your plan for the week ahead in whatever format you wish.

Monday	Tuesday	Wednesday
Thursday	**Friday**	**Saturday**

Monday- Date: _____	
My Morning Wellbeing Check-In || **Morning Prompts**

My Morning Wellbeing Check-In		Morning Prompts
Sleep ☆☆☆☆☆	Energy Levels ☆☆☆☆☆	1. What three things can I do today that will make me feel it was a great day when I reflect before I go to sleep?
Mood ☆☆☆☆☆	Muscle Soreness ☆☆☆☆☆	2. What relationships would I like to strengthen today and how can I do this?
Total Wellbeing Score		3. Something I've been putting off that I can do today is...

Morning Challenge- Return to page 9 and read your personal definition of *Commitment* three times.

My Evening Wellbeing Markers		Evening Prompts
Hydration ☆☆☆☆☆	Nutrition ☆☆☆☆☆	1. What did I do well today and why/how?
Daylight/Outside ☆☆☆☆☆	Phone ☆☆☆☆☆	2. What is currently bringing energy to my life?
Total Wellbeing Score		3. What is currently draining me and what can I do to overcome this?
Tick here when you have completed your habit/action/metric *tracker*.		

Tuesday- Date: _____			
My Morning Wellbeing Check-In		**Morning Prompts**	
Sleep ☆☆☆☆☆	Energy Levels ☆☆☆☆☆	1. What three things can I do today that will make me feel it was a great day when I reflect before I go to sleep?	
Mood ☆☆☆☆☆	Muscle Soreness ☆☆☆☆☆	2. How can I add more fun to my day today?	
Total Wellbeing Score		3. List three benefits of journaling, planning and tracking.	

....
....
....
....
....
....
....
....
....
....
....
....
....
....
....

Morning Challenge- Rewrite your personal definition of *Commitment* from memory and then return to page 9 to check for accuracy. Give it your best shot. Don't expect it to be perfect. It doesn't need to be.

....
....
....
....

My Evening Wellbeing Markers		Evening Prompts
Hydration ☆☆☆☆☆	Nutrition ☆☆☆☆☆	1. Write about one great moment from today in detail.
Daylight/Outside ☆☆☆☆☆	Phone ☆☆☆☆☆	2. In general, what is something that makes you feel knocked off course, reactive, and not at your personal best? Why do you feel this is so?
Total Wellbeing Score		3. It's hard for me to open up about...
Tick here when you have completed your habit/action/metric *tracker*.		

Wednesday- Date: _____			
My Morning Wellbeing Check-In			**Morning Prompts**
Sleep ☆☆☆☆☆		Energy Levels ☆☆☆☆☆	1. What three things can I do today that will make me feel it was a great day when I reflect before I go to sleep?
Mood ☆☆☆☆☆		Muscle Soreness ☆☆☆☆☆	2. What can I do today to make me feel more connected to other people?
Total Wellbeing Score			3. I would feel lighter if I let go of…

Morning Challenge- Return to page 9 and read your personal definition of *Success* three times.

My Evening Wellbeing Markers		Evening Journaling
Hydration ☆☆☆☆☆	Nutrition ☆☆☆☆☆	This is a *Stream of Consciousness Journaling* type of challenge. Simply write down all that comes to your mind below. There is no required outcome here, only to let whatever needs to come out... out. Write for ten minutes and use the blank pages provided at the back if necessary. Just... write!
Daylight/Outside ☆☆☆☆☆	Phone ☆☆☆☆☆	
Total Wellbeing Score		
Tick here when you have completed your habit/action/metric *tracker*.		

Thursday- Date: _____			
My Morning Wellbeing Check-In			**Morning Prompts**
Sleep ☆☆☆☆☆		Energy Levels ☆☆☆☆☆	1. What three things can I do today that will make me feel it was a great day when I reflect before I go to sleep?
Mood ☆☆☆☆☆		Muscle Soreness ☆☆☆☆☆	2. What would it look like for me to live true to my values today?
Total Wellbeing Score			3. Today I want to use the best of my energy to...

Morning Challenge- Rewrite your personal definition of *Success* from memory and then return to page 9 to check for accuracy. Give it your best shot. Don't expect it to be perfect. It doesn't need to be.

My Evening Wellbeing Markers		Evening Prompts
Hydration ☆☆☆☆☆	Nutrition ☆☆☆☆☆	1. What could I have done better today and what are the lessons to be learned from this?
Daylight/Outside ☆☆☆☆☆	Phone ☆☆☆☆☆	2. What is making me proud?
Total Wellbeing Score		3. What intrigues me? What am I curious about?
Tick here when you have completed your habit/action/metric *tracker*.		

Friday- Date: _____			
My Morning Wellbeing Check-In			**Morning Prompts**
Sleep ☆☆☆☆☆	Energy Levels ☆☆☆☆☆		1. What three things can I do today that will make me feel it was a great day when I reflect before I go to sleep?
Mood ☆☆☆☆☆	Muscle Soreness ☆☆☆☆☆		2. How can I make those around me feel special today?
Total Wellbeing Score			3. I am excited about…

My Evening Wellbeing Markers		Evening Prompts
Hydration ☆☆☆☆☆	Nutrition ☆☆☆☆☆	1. How do you feel you are influencing others in a positive way?
Daylight/Outside ☆☆☆☆☆	Phone ☆☆☆☆☆	2. What did I learn or relearn today?
Total Wellbeing Score		3. For me happiness is to be found...
Tick here when you have completed your habit/action/metric *tracker*.		

Saturday- Date: _____
Time to Reflect and Summarise My Learnings

My Weekly Wellbeing Check-In Averages				
Sleep ☆☆☆☆☆	Energy Levels ☆☆☆☆☆	Hydration ☆☆☆☆☆	Nutrition ☆☆☆☆☆
Mood ☆☆☆☆☆	Muscle Soreness ☆☆☆☆☆	Daylight/Outside ☆☆☆☆☆	Phone ☆☆☆☆☆
My Average Wellness Score			
Out of 5, rate your consistency in using your habit/action/metric tracker			

Based on these scores, I need to:

Start _____

Stop _____

Continue _____

Your challenge is to complete five of these prompts at the very least; maybe more and perhaps even all of them. Simply write the number of the prompt and journal your response in the space provided. This is important work!

1) Note one example of how you lived according to your values/personal mission statement this week and explain how this made you feel.
2) Describe one way your values/personal mission statement were challenged or compromised this week and explain what you learned from this experience.
3) List two things that went well this week inside or outside of sport and offer reasons as to why.
4) What were your two most important learnings or relearnings this week (one inside sport and one outside of sport) and explain how you plan to bring these forward to better yourself?
5) What did you come across this week that you were interested in or were curious about, and would like to look into at a deeper level? How or where can you learn more about this?
6) Think of an example from the past week where you were *fully engaged*. Explain in detail how it felt to be *fully engaged*.
7) What relationships did I improve this week and how?
8) Who helped you this week and how?
9) I was a good teammate this week because...
10) I improved as an athlete this week by...
11) One great moment from the week I want to remember is...
12) My top three accomplishments from the week were:
13) Write a note on the progress you have made this week with regard to achieving your goals.
14) My key takeaways from this week are:

My Four-Week Review

Date: _____

Review your habit/action/metric *tracker* for this four-week block:
1. List the areas where you have shown consistency and progress.
2. List the areas you would like to show more consistency over the next period.

Review your *Wellness Scores* for the past four Saturdays. Based on these scores, I need to:

Start

Stop

Continue

Review your past four weeks journaling, in particular your Saturdays, and …

Select your top two learnings or relearnings from this period.

Select your top two accomplishments from this period.

Select the top two ways you have improved as an athlete over this period.

Select your top two takeaways from this period.

My Next Four Weeks

My Learning Tools

My Learning Tools

My Learning Tools

My Learning Tools

My Goals – My Intentions

Signed: _____ Date: _____

My Goals – My Intentions

Signed: _____ Date: _____

My Tracker

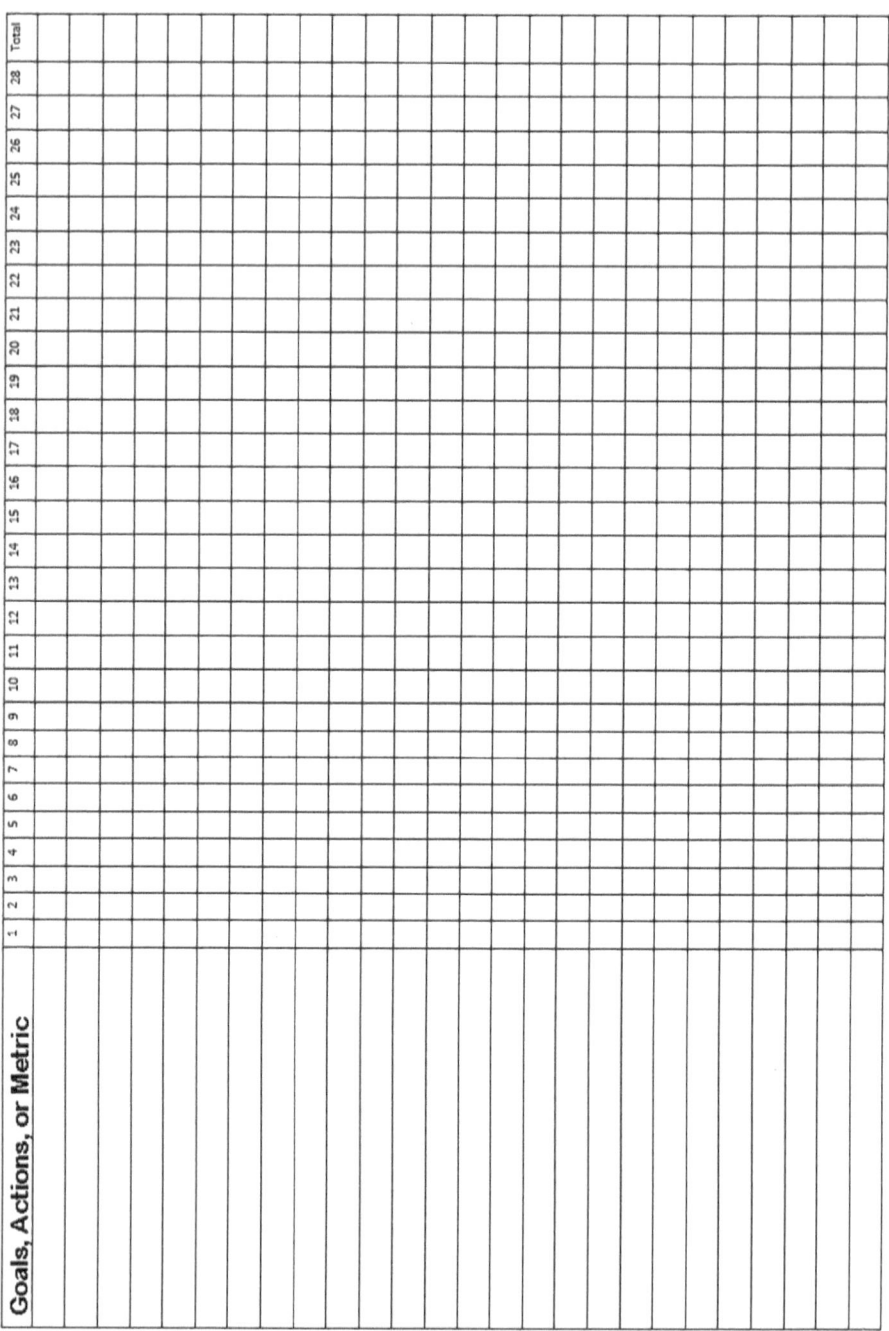

My Next Four Weeks – Important Things

(You can fill in the date in the small boxes provided in the top left-hand corner.)

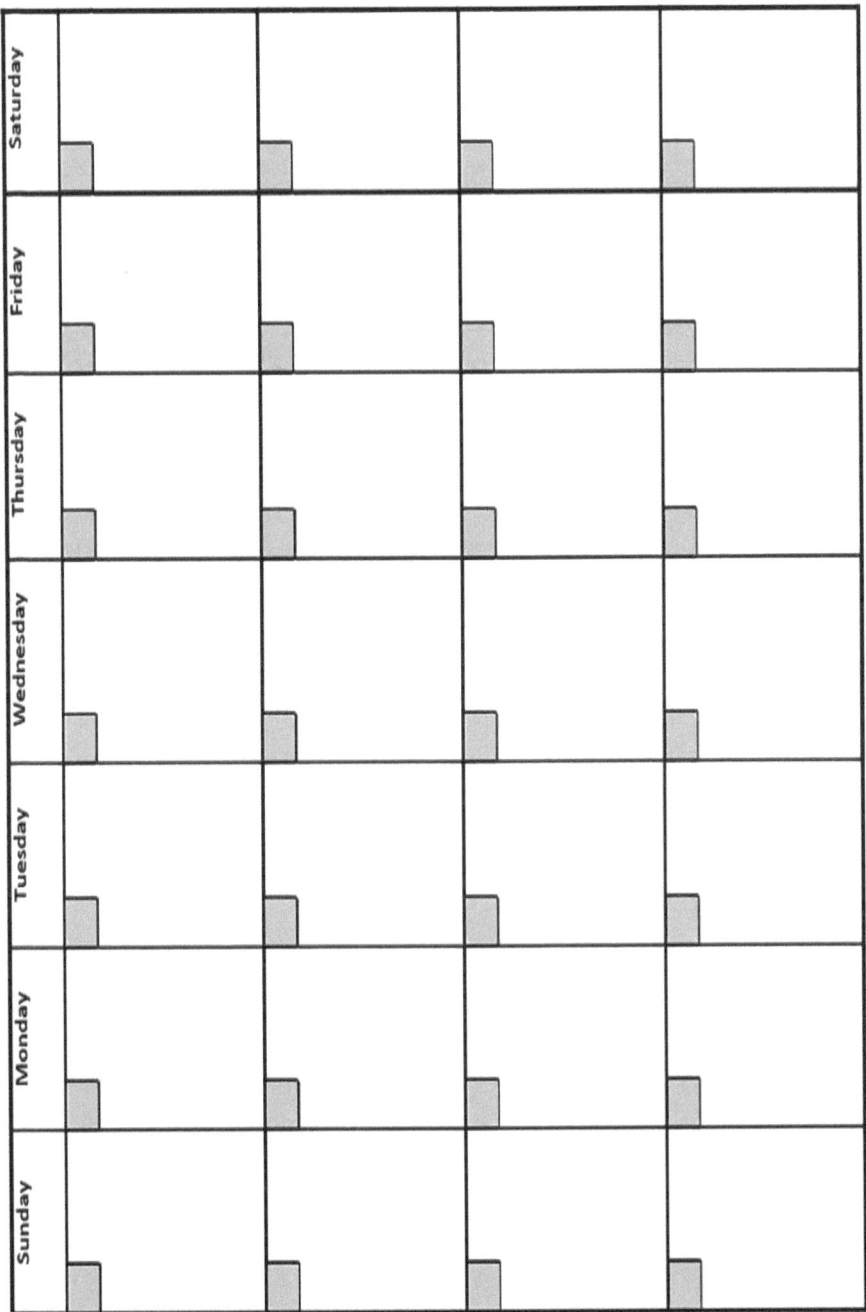

Sunday- Time to Plan for the Week Ahead

Date: _____

Your challenge is to complete three of these prompts at the very least; maybe more and perhaps even all of them. Simply write the number of the prompt and journal your response in the space provided. This is important work!

1) Describe in detail how you intend to live this week. Here you may wish to draw insights from your Values, your *Personal Mission Statement*, and your goals or intentions.
2) List at least one area of your life outside of sport that you would like to live with intention this week and explain the behaviours or actions required to do so.
3) Describe in detail at least one way you are going to improve as a teammate this week and explain how that will make you feel.
4) Describe in detail how you plan to improve as an athlete this week: what tools and practices are you going to utilise, what are your key *work-ons*, who or what can help you, etc.
5) What are the biggest sporting challenges that lay ahead of you this week? How to do want to 'show up' for these?
6) Full engagement is the acquired ability to give your full and best energy and effort to what you are doing at any given moment. Where is the one area you would like to be *fully engaged* this week and why is it important you do so?
7) In order to bring balance, recreation, regeneration and joy to your life this week what hobbies, interests or activities outside of sport do you need to make time for?
8) To help me make progress towards achieving my goals or living my intentions, this week I will…(List five actions.)

_____
_____
_____
_____
_____
_____
_____
_____
_____
_____
_____
_____

Important for the Week Ahead

Here you can use the blank spaces to schedule or craft your plan for the week ahead in whatever format you wish.

Monday	Tuesday	Wednesday

Thursday	Friday	Saturday

Monday- Date: _____			
My Morning Wellbeing Check-In			**Morning Prompts**
Sleep ☆☆☆☆☆	Energy Levels ☆☆☆☆☆		1. What am I grateful for this morning? Explain in detail.
Mood ☆☆☆☆☆	Muscle Soreness ☆☆☆☆☆		2. How do I want to feel today and what am I willing to do to achieve this?
Total Wellbeing Score			3. I will smile when my head hits the pillow this evening if…

_____

Morning Challenge- Return to page 5 and read your *Values* and their definitions three times.

My Evening Wellbeing Markers		Evening Prompts
Hydration ☆☆☆☆☆	Nutrition ☆☆☆☆☆	1. What did I do well today and why/how?
Daylight/Outside ☆☆☆☆☆	Phone ☆☆☆☆☆	2. What did I learn or relearn today?
Total Wellbeing Score		3. What is one thing I could have done better today and how?
Tick here when you have completed your habit/action/metric *tracker*.		

Tuesday- Date: _____			
My Morning Wellbeing Check-In			**Morning Prompts**
Sleep ☆☆☆☆☆	Energy Levels ☆☆☆☆☆		1. What am I grateful for this morning? Explain in detail.
Mood ☆☆☆☆☆	Muscle Soreness ☆☆☆☆☆		2. Who would I like to connect with today and why?
Total Wellbeing Score			3. What can I do in order to inject more fun into the day ahead?

Morning Challenge- Return to page 5 and read your *Values* and their definitions three times.

My Evening Wellbeing Markers		Evening Prompts
Hydration ☆☆☆☆☆	Nutrition ☆☆☆☆☆	1. What were the three best things about today?
Daylight/Outside ☆☆☆☆☆	Phone ☆☆☆☆☆	2. Who did I help today, how did I help them and how did it make me feel? Who could I have helped more?
Total Wellbeing Score		3. Something I am procrastinating over is... What action should I take?
Tick here when you have completed your habit/action/metric *tracker*.		

Wednesday- Date: _____

My Morning Wellbeing Check-In		Morning Prompts
Sleep ☆☆☆☆☆	Energy Levels ☆☆☆☆☆	1. What am I grateful for this morning? Explain in detail.
Mood ☆☆☆☆☆	Muscle Soreness ☆☆☆☆☆	2. Write about a positive experience from yesterday: what was it, why did it come about and how did it make you feel?
Total Wellbeing Score		3. I feel good when I start my day with….

Morning Challenge- Rewrite your *Values* and their definitions from memory and then return to page 5 to check for accuracy. Give it your best shot. Don't expect it to be perfect. It doesn't need to be.

My Evening Wellbeing Markers		Evening Journaling
Hydration ☆☆☆☆☆	Nutrition ☆☆☆☆☆	This is a *Stream of Consciousness Journaling* type of challenge. Simply write down all that comes to your mind below. There is no required outcome here, only to let whatever needs to come out... out. Write for ten minutes and use the blank pages provided at the back if necessary. Just... write!
Daylight/Outside ☆☆☆☆☆	Phone ☆☆☆☆☆	
Total Wellbeing Score		
Tick here when you have completed your habit/action/metric *tracker*.		

Thursday- Date: _____			
My Morning Wellbeing Check-In			**Morning Prompts**
Sleep ☆☆☆☆☆	Energy Levels ☆☆☆☆☆		1. What am I grateful for this morning? Explain in detail.
Mood ☆☆☆☆☆	Muscle Soreness ☆☆☆☆☆		2. What precisely is adding energy to my life right now?
Total Wellbeing Score			3. What is one thing I can do today to bring more happiness into my day?

Morning Challenge- Read your *Personal Mission Statement* from page 6 three times.

My Evening Wellbeing Markers		Evening Prompts
Hydration ☆☆☆☆☆	Nutrition ☆☆☆☆☆	1. Write about the highlight of your day; think- what, why, when, where, who and how.
Daylight/Outside ☆☆☆☆☆	Phone ☆☆☆☆☆	2. What did I learn or relearn today?
Total Wellbeing Score		3. How did I grow as an athlete and person today?
Tick here when you have completed your habit/action/metric *tracker*.		

Friday- Date: _____		
My Morning Wellbeing Check-In		**Morning Prompts**
Sleep ☆☆☆☆☆	Energy Levels ☆☆☆☆☆	1. What am I grateful for this morning? Explain in detail.
Mood ☆☆☆☆☆	Muscle Soreness ☆☆☆☆☆	2. As I look towards the day ahead write down: two things I can control, two things I can influence and two things I can't control.
Total Wellbeing Score		3 What three things are most important for me today and how can I tend to these?

Morning Challenge- Rewrite your *Personal Mission Statement* from memory and then return to page 6 to check for accuracy. Give it your best shot. Don't expect it to be perfect. It doesn't need to be.

My Evening Wellbeing Markers		Evening Prompts
Hydration ☆☆☆☆☆	Nutrition ☆☆☆☆☆	1. What is currently bringing the most joy to my life and why?
Daylight/Outside ☆☆☆☆☆	Phone ☆☆☆☆☆	2. My greatest learning resources as an athlete are... (think: who, what, where, how).
Total Wellbeing Score		3. I live true to my values when I...
Tick here when you have completed your habit/action/metric *tracker*.		

Saturday- Date: _____
Time to Reflect and Summarise My Learnings

My Weekly Wellbeing Check-In Averages			
Sleep ☆☆☆☆☆	Energy Levels ☆☆☆☆☆	Hydration ☆☆☆☆☆	Nutrition ☆☆☆☆☆
Mood ☆☆☆☆☆	Muscle Soreness ☆☆☆☆☆	Daylight/Outside ☆☆☆☆☆	Phone ☆☆☆☆☆
My Average Wellness Score			
Out of 5, rate your consistency in using your habit/action/metric *tracker*			

Based on these scores, I need to:

Start _____

Stop _____

Continue _____

Your challenge is to complete five of these prompts at the very least; maybe more and perhaps even all of them. Simply write the number of the prompt and journal your response in the space provided. This is important work!

1) Note one example of how you lived according to your values/personal mission statement this week and explain how this made you feel.
2) Describe one way your values/personal mission statement were challenged or compromised this week and explain what you learned from this experience.
3) List two things that went well this week inside or outside of sport and offer reasons as to why.
4) What were your two most important learnings or relearnings this week (one inside sport and one outside of sport) and explain how you plan to bring these forward to better yourself?
5) What did you come across this week that you were interested in or were curious about, and would like to look into at a deeper level? How or where can you learn more about this?
6) Think of an example from the past week where you were *fully engaged*. Explain in detail how it felt to be *fully engaged*.
7) What relationships did I improve this week and how?
8) Who helped you this week and how?
9) I was a good teammate this week because…
10) I improved as an athlete this week by…
11) One great moment from the week I want to remember is…
12) My top three accomplishments from the week were:
13) Write a note on the progress you have made this week with regard to achieving your goals.
14) My key takeaways from this week are:

Sunday- Time to Plan for the Week Ahead

Date: _____

Your challenge is to complete three of these prompts at the very least; maybe more and perhaps even all of them. Simply write the number of the prompt and journal your response in the space provided. This is important work!

1) Describe in detail how you intend to live this week. Here you may wish to draw insights from your Values, your *Personal Mission Statement*, and your goals or intentions.
2) List at least one area of your life outside of sport that you would like to live with intention this week and explain the behaviours or actions required to do so.
3) Describe in detail at least one way you are going to improve as a teammate this week and explain how that will make you feel.
4) Describe in detail how you plan to improve as an athlete this week: what tools and practices are you going to utilise, what are your key *work-ons*, who or what can help you, etc.
5) What are the biggest sporting challenges that lay ahead of you this week? How to do want to 'show up' for these?
6) Full engagement is the acquired ability to give your full and best energy and effort to what you are doing at any given moment. Where is the one area you would like to be *fully engaged* this week and why is it important you do so?
7) In order to bring balance, recreation, regeneration and joy to your life this week what hobbies, interests or activities outside of sport do you need to make time for?
8) To help me make progress towards achieving my goals or living my intentions, this week I will…(List five actions.)

Important for the Week Ahead

Here you can use the blank spaces to schedule or craft your plan for the week ahead in whatever format you wish.

Monday	Tuesday	Wednesday

Thursday	Friday	Saturday

Monday- Date: _____			
My Morning Wellbeing Check-In			**Morning Prompts**
Sleep ☆☆☆☆☆	Energy Levels ☆☆☆☆☆		1. List three things that are good about today.
Mood ☆☆☆☆☆	Muscle Soreness ☆☆☆☆☆		2. Write the names of three people you interact with daily. Note at least one positive thing about each of them.
Total Wellbeing Score			3. How can I be kind to myself today?

Morning Challenge- Return to page 6 and read your explanation of, or answer to, 'What Sport Means to Me' three times.

My Evening Wellbeing Markers		Evening Prompts
Hydration ☆☆☆☆☆	Nutrition ☆☆☆☆☆	1. What is currently bringing satisfaction into my life?
Daylight/Outside ☆☆☆☆☆	Phone ☆☆☆☆☆	2. Where in my life am I currently making excuses? How can I improve this?
Total Wellbeing Score		3. I feel good when I end my day with…
Tick here when you have completed your habit/action/metric *tracker*.		

Tuesday- Date: _____			
My Morning Wellbeing Check-In			**Morning Prompts**
Sleep ☆☆☆☆☆	Energy Levels ☆☆☆☆☆		1. List three things that are good about today.
Mood ☆☆☆☆☆	Muscle Soreness ☆☆☆☆☆		2. Who am I when I am at my very best (physically, mentally, spiritually, etc.)? Write between six to ten words that you believe are representative of you when you're most proud of yourself, regardless of circumstance or situation.
Total Wellbeing Score			3. Why is it important to be my authentic self?

_____
_____
_____
_____
_____
_____
_____
_____
_____
_____
_____
_____

Morning Challenge- Rewrite 'What Sport Means to Me' from memory and then return to page 6 to check for accuracy. Give it your best shot. Don't expect it to be perfect. It doesn't need to be.

_____
_____
_____
_____
_____
_____

My Evening Wellbeing Markers		Evening Prompts
Hydration ☆☆☆☆☆	Nutrition ☆☆☆☆☆	1. Three ways I was true to my *Values* today:
Daylight/Outside ☆☆☆☆☆	Phone ☆☆☆☆☆	2. List and explain at least two ways you feel like you are influencing others in a positive way.
Total Wellbeing Score		3. I am proud of myself today because…
Tick here when you have completed your habit/action/metric *tracker*.		

Wednesday- Date: _____			
My Morning Wellbeing Check-In			**Morning Prompts**
Sleep ☆☆☆☆☆		Energy Levels ☆☆☆☆☆	1. List three things that are good about today.
Mood ☆☆☆☆☆		Muscle Soreness ☆☆☆☆☆	2. What three things can I do today that will make me feel it was a great day when I reflect before I go to sleep?
Total Wellbeing Score			3. What is my most important 'Value' and why?

Morning Challenge- Return to page 7 and read your explanation for, or answer to, 'My Vision for Myself as a Teammate' three times.

My Evening Wellbeing Markers		Evening Journaling
Hydration ☆☆☆☆☆	Nutrition ☆☆☆☆☆	This is a *Stream of Consciousness Journaling* type of challenge. Simply write down all that comes to your mind below. There is no required outcome here, only to let whatever needs to come out… out. Write for ten minutes and use the blank pages provided at the back if necessary. Just… write!
Daylight/Outside ☆☆☆☆☆	Phone ☆☆☆☆☆	
Total Wellbeing Score		
Tick here when you have completed your habit/action/metric *tracker*.		

Thursday- Date: _____			
My Morning Wellbeing Check-In			**Morning Prompts**
Sleep ☆☆☆☆☆		Energy Levels ☆☆☆☆☆	1. List three things that are good about today.
Mood ☆☆☆☆☆		Muscle Soreness ☆☆☆☆☆	2. Write up a rough plan for the day ahead. Include the major events in your day and note how you wish to turn up and present yourself in each of these situations.
Total Wellbeing Score			3. Today I will…

_____

Morning Challenge- Rewrite your 'My Vision for Myself as a Teammate' from memory and then return to page 7 to check for accuracy. Give it your best shot. Don't expect it to be perfect. It doesn't need to be.

_____

My Evening Wellbeing Markers		Evening Prompts
Hydration ☆☆☆☆☆	Nutrition ☆☆☆☆☆	1. List three things that were good about today.
Daylight/Outside ☆☆☆☆☆	Phone ☆☆☆☆☆	2. Describe your biggest learning or relearning from today.
Total Wellbeing Score		3. Who helped me today and how did they help me?
Tick here when you have completed your habit/action/metric *tracker*.		

Friday- Date: _____			
My Morning Wellbeing Check-In			**Morning Prompts**
Sleep ☆☆☆☆☆		Energy Levels ☆☆☆☆☆	1. List three things that are good about today.
Mood ☆☆☆☆☆		Muscle Soreness ☆☆☆☆☆	2. How/Where/To whom do I want to show kindness today?
Total Wellbeing Score			3 What three things are most important to me for the day ahead?

My Evening Wellbeing Markers		Evening Prompts
Hydration ☆☆☆☆☆	Nutrition ☆☆☆☆☆	1. What did I do well today and why/how?
Daylight/Outside ☆☆☆☆☆	Phone ☆☆☆☆☆	2. Return to this morning's journal prompt where you were asked to list three things you felt were most important for you for the day ahead. Did you tend to these things in a satisfactory manner? If the answer is Yes: explain how this makes you feel. If the answer is No: explain your strongest reason for not doing it.
Total Wellbeing Score		3. What are the habits, behaviours or distractions that pull me away from being present or in the moment?
Tick here when you have completed your habit/action/metric *tracker*.		

Saturday- Date: _____			
Time to Reflect and Summarise My Learnings			
My Weekly Wellbeing Check-In Averages			
Sleep ☆☆☆☆☆	Energy Levels ☆☆☆☆☆	Hydration ☆☆☆☆☆	Nutrition ☆☆☆☆☆
Mood ☆☆☆☆☆	Muscle Soreness ☆☆☆☆☆	Daylight/Outside ☆☆☆☆☆	Phone ☆☆☆☆☆
My Average Wellness Score			
Out of 5, rate your consistency in using your habit/action/metric tracker			

Based on these scores, I need to:

Start

Stop

Continue

Your challenge is to complete five of these prompts at the very least; maybe more and perhaps even all of them. Simply write the number of the prompt and journal your response in the space provided. This is important work!

1) Note one example of how you lived according to your values/personal mission statement this week and explain how this made you feel.
2) Describe one way your values/personal mission statement were challenged or compromised this week and explain what you learned from this experience.
3) List two things that went well this week inside or outside of sport and offer reasons as to why.
4) What were your two most important learnings or relearnings this week (one inside sport and one outside of sport) and explain how you plan to bring these forward to better yourself?
5) What did you come across this week that you were interested in or were curious about, and would like to look into at a deeper level? How or where can you learn more about this?
6) Think of an example from the past week where you were *fully engaged*. Explain in detail how it felt to be *fully engaged*.
7) What relationships did I improve this week and how?
8) Who helped you this week and how?
9) I was a good teammate this week because…
10) I improved as an athlete this week by…
11) One great moment from the week I want to remember is…
12) My top three accomplishments from the week were:
13) Write a note on the progress you have made this week with regard to achieving your goals.
14) My key takeaways from this week are:

Sunday- Time to Plan for the Week Ahead

Date: _____

Your challenge is to complete three of these prompts at the very least; maybe more and perhaps even all of them. Simply write the number of the prompt and journal your response in the space provided. This is important work!

1) Describe in detail how you intend to live this week. Here you may wish to draw insights from your Values, your *Personal Mission Statement*, and your goals or intentions.
2) List at least one area of your life outside of sport that you would like to live with intention this week and explain the behaviours or actions required to do so.
3) Describe in detail at least one way you are going to improve as a teammate this week and explain how that will make you feel.
4) Describe in detail how you plan to improve as an athlete this week: what tools and practices are you going to utilise, what are your key *work-ons*, who or what can help you, etc.
5) What are the biggest sporting challenges that lay ahead of you this week? How to do want to 'show up' for these?
6) Full engagement is the acquired ability to give your full and best energy and effort to what you are doing at any given moment. Where is the one area you would like to be *fully engaged* this week and why is it important you do so?
7) In order to bring balance, recreation, regeneration and joy to your life this week what hobbies, interests or activities outside of sport do you need to make time for?
8) To help me make progress towards achieving my goals or living my intentions, this week I will…(List five actions.)

Important for the Week Ahead

Here you can use the blank spaces to schedule or craft your plan for the week ahead in whatever format you wish.

Monday	Tuesday	Wednesday

Thursday	Friday	Saturday

Monday- Date: _____

My Morning Wellbeing Check-In		Morning Prompts
Sleep ☆☆☆☆☆	Energy Levels ☆☆☆☆☆	1. Complete this sentence three times: I am grateful for … because…
Mood ☆☆☆☆☆	Muscle Soreness ☆☆☆☆☆	2. Name one area you would like to be *fully engaged* today and explain why. We will refer to it this evening as your *fully engaged target area*.
Total Wellbeing Score		3. Write down some core principles for the day- What principles do I want to live by today?

_____

Morning Challenge- Return to page 8 and read your explanation of, or answer to, 'My truth or belief around application to collective and individual practice' three times.

My Evening Wellbeing Markers		Evening Prompts
Hydration ☆☆☆☆☆	Nutrition ☆☆☆☆☆	1. How did your *fully engaged target area* from this morning play out for you? What lessons did you learn?
Daylight/Outside ☆☆☆☆☆	Phone ☆☆☆☆☆	2. Where have I been doing well of late? In what areas have I been growing?
Total Wellbeing Score		3. What am I currently finding inspiring?
Tick here when you have completed your habit/action/metric *tracker*.		

Tuesday- Date: _____			
My Morning Wellbeing Check-In			**Morning Prompts**
Sleep ☆☆☆☆☆		Energy Levels ☆☆☆☆☆	1. Complete this sentence three times: I am grateful for ... because...
Mood ☆☆☆☆☆		Muscle Soreness ☆☆☆☆☆	2. Describe how you can behave and prepare like a champion today.
Total Wellbeing Score			3. Finish the following- I am... I can... I will...

_____
_____
_____
_____
_____
_____
_____
_____
_____
_____
_____
_____
_____
_____

Morning Challenge- Rewrite your 'My truth or belief around application to collective and individual practice' from memory and then return to page 8 to check for accuracy. Give it your best shot. Don't expect it to be perfect. It doesn't need to be.

_____
_____
_____
_____

My Evening Wellbeing Markers		Evening Prompts
Hydration ☆☆☆☆	Nutrition ☆☆☆☆☆	1. Champions consistently make good choices. Make a list of 'champion choices'.
Daylight/Outside ☆☆☆☆☆	Phone ☆☆☆☆☆	2. What did I learn or relearn today?
Total Wellbeing Score		3. Write about an area in your life where you feel stuck right now and how you can begin to make progress here.
Tick here when you have completed your habit/action/metric *tracker*.		

Wednesday- Date: _____			
My Morning Wellbeing Check-In		**Morning Prompts**	
Sleep ☆☆☆☆☆	Energy Levels ☆☆☆☆☆	1. Complete this sentence three times: I am grateful for ... because...	
Mood ☆☆☆☆☆	Muscle Soreness ☆☆☆☆☆	2. How can I have a positive impact on others today?	
Total Wellbeing Score		3. Today I will nourish my body and mind by...	

Morning Challenge- Return to page 9 and read your personal definition of *Excellence* three times.

My Evening Wellbeing Markers		Evening Journaling
Hydration ☆☆☆☆☆	Nutrition ☆☆☆☆☆	This is a *Stream of Consciousness Journaling* type of challenge. Simply write down all that comes to your mind below. There is no required outcome here, only to let whatever needs to come out... out. Write for ten minutes and use the blank pages provided at the back if necessary. Just... write!
Daylight/Outside ☆☆☆☆☆	Phone ☆☆☆☆☆	
Total Wellbeing Score		
Tick here when you have completed your habit/action/metric *tracker*.		

Thursday- Date: _____

My Morning Wellbeing Check-In		Morning Prompts
Sleep ☆☆☆☆☆	Energy Levels ☆☆☆☆☆	1. Complete this sentence three times: I am grateful for ... because...
Mood ☆☆☆☆☆	Muscle Soreness ☆☆☆☆☆	2. Write for five minutes... 'I feel happiest when...' let it flow.
Total Wellbeing Score		3. How do I plan to grow as an athlete and person today?

Morning Challenge - Rewrite your personal definition of *Excellence* from memory and then return to page 9 to check for accuracy. Give it your best shot. Don't expect it to be perfect. It doesn't need to be.

My Evening Wellbeing Markers		Evening Prompts
Hydration ☆☆☆☆☆	Nutrition ☆☆☆☆☆	1. Much of sport involves dealing with discomfort, challenge and pressure. Write out a clear vision of how you want to show up in times of discomfort, challenge, and pressure. Take your time here; go deep, bring clarity.
Daylight/Outside ☆☆☆☆☆	Phone ☆☆☆☆☆	2. Where am I making real progress and why?
Total Wellbeing Score		3. I can add more depth to my life by…
Tick here when you have completed your habit/action/metric *tracker*.		

Friday- Date: _____

My Morning Wellbeing Check-In		Morning Prompts
Sleep ☆☆☆☆☆	Energy Levels ☆☆☆☆☆	1. Complete this sentence three times: I am grateful for … because…
Mood ☆☆☆☆☆	Muscle Soreness ☆☆☆☆☆	2. Explain how you can bring your values into your interactions and experiences today.
Total Wellbeing Score		3. I find meaning and purpose in…

My Evening Wellbeing Markers		Evening Prompts
Hydration ☆☆☆☆☆	Nutrition ☆☆☆☆☆	1. What do I need to do more of and why?
Daylight/Outside ☆☆☆☆☆	Phone ☆☆☆☆☆	2. What do I need to do less of and why?
Total Wellbeing Score		3. What do I need to keep doing and why?
Tick here when you have completed your habit/action/metric *tracker*.		

Saturday- Date: _____			
Time to Reflect and Summarise My Learnings			
My Weekly Wellbeing Check-In Averages			
Sleep ☆☆☆☆☆	Energy Levels ☆☆☆☆☆	Hydration ☆☆☆☆☆	Nutrition ☆☆☆☆☆
Mood ☆☆☆☆☆	Muscle Soreness ☆☆☆☆☆	Daylight/Outside ☆☆☆☆☆	Phone ☆☆☆☆☆
My Average Wellness Score			
Out of 5, rate your consistency in using your habit/action/metric tracker			

Based on these scores, I need to:

Start _____

Stop _____

Continue _____

Your challenge is to complete five of these prompts at the very least; maybe more and perhaps even all of them. Simply write the number of the prompt and journal your response in the space provided. This is important work!

1) Note one example of how you lived according to your values/personal mission statement this week and explain how this made you feel.
2) Describe one way your values/personal mission statement were challenged or compromised this week and explain what you learned from this experience.
3) List two things that went well this week inside or outside of sport and offer reasons as to why.
4) What were your two most important learnings or relearnings this week (one inside sport and one outside of sport) and explain how you plan to bring these forward to better yourself?
5) What did you come across this week that you were interested in or were curious about, and would like to look into at a deeper level? How or where can you learn more about this?
6) Think of an example from the past week where you were *fully engaged*. Explain in detail how it felt to be *fully engaged*.
7) What relationships did I improve this week and how?
8) Who helped you this week and how?
9) I was a good teammate this week because...
10) I improved as an athlete this week by...
11) One great moment from the week I want to remember is...
12) My top three accomplishments from the week were:
13) Write a note on the progress you have made this week with regard to achieving your goals.
14) My key takeaways from this week are:

Sunday- Time to Plan for the Week Ahead

Date: _____

Your challenge is to complete three of these prompts at the very least; maybe more and perhaps even all of them. Simply write the number of the prompt and journal your response in the space provided. This is important work!

1) Describe in detail how you intend to live this week. Here you may wish to draw insights from your Values, your *Personal Mission Statement*, and your goals or intentions.
2) List at least one area of your life outside of sport that you would like to live with intention this week and explain the behaviours or actions required to do so.
3) Describe in detail at least one way you are going to improve as a teammate this week and explain how that will make you feel.
4) Describe in detail how you plan to improve as an athlete this week: what tools and practices are you going to utilise, what are your key *work-ons*, who or what can help you, etc.
5) What are the biggest sporting challenges that lay ahead of you this week? How to do want to 'show up' for these?
6) Full engagement is the acquired ability to give your full and best energy and effort to what you are doing at any given moment. Where is the one area you would like to be *fully engaged* this week and why is it important you do so?
7) In order to bring balance, recreation, regeneration and joy to your life this week what hobbies, interests or activities outside of sport do you need to make time for?
8) To help me make progress towards achieving my goals or living my intentions, this week I will...(List five actions.)

Important for the Week Ahead

Here you can use the blank spaces to schedule or craft your plan for the week ahead in whatever format you wish.

Monday	Tuesday	Wednesday
Thursday	**Friday**	**Saturday**

Monday- Date: _____			
My Morning Wellbeing Check-In			**Morning Prompts**
Sleep ☆☆☆☆☆	Energy Levels ☆☆☆☆☆		1. What three things can I do today that will make me feel it was a great day when I reflect before I go to sleep?
Mood ☆☆☆☆☆	Muscle Soreness ☆☆☆☆☆		2. What relationships would I like to strengthen today and how can I do this?
Total Wellbeing Score			3. Something I've been putting off that I can do today is...

Morning Challenge- Return to page 9 and read your personal definition of *Commitment* three times.

My Evening Wellbeing Markers		Evening Prompts
Hydration ☆☆☆☆☆	Nutrition ☆☆☆☆☆	1. What did I do well today and why/how?
Daylight/Outside ☆☆☆☆☆	Phone ☆☆☆☆☆	2. What is currently bringing energy to my life?
Total Wellbeing Score		3. What is currently draining me and what can I do to overcome this?
Tick here when you have completed your habit/action/metric *tracker*.		

Tuesday- Date: _____			
My Morning Wellbeing Check-In			**Morning Prompts**
Sleep ☆☆☆☆☆	Energy Levels ☆☆☆☆☆		1. What three things can I do today that will make me feel it was a great day when I reflect before I go to sleep?
Mood ☆☆☆☆☆	Muscle Soreness ☆☆☆☆☆		2. How can I add more fun to my day today?
Total Wellbeing Score			3. List three benefits of journaling, planning and tracking.

Morning Challenge- Rewrite your personal definition of *Commitment* from memory and then return to page 9 to check for accuracy. Give it your best shot. Don't expect it to be perfect. It doesn't need to be.

My Evening Wellbeing Markers		Evening Prompts
Hydration ☆☆☆☆☆	Nutrition ☆☆☆☆☆	1. Write about one great moment from today in detail.
Daylight/Outside ☆☆☆☆☆	Phone ☆☆☆☆☆	2. In general, what is something that makes you feel knocked off course, reactive, and not at your personal best? Why do you feel this is so?
Total Wellbeing Score		3. It's hard for me to open up about…
Tick here when you have completed your habit/action/metric *tracker*.		

Wednesday- Date: _____			
My Morning Wellbeing Check-In		**Morning Prompts**	
Sleep ☆☆☆☆☆	Energy Levels ☆☆☆☆☆	1. What three things can I do today that will make me feel it was a great day when I reflect before I go to sleep?	
Mood ☆☆☆☆☆	Muscle Soreness ☆☆☆☆☆	2. What can I do today to make me feel more connected to other people?	
Total Wellbeing Score		3. I would feel lighter if I let go of…	

Morning Challenge- Return to page 9 and read your personal definition of *Success* three times.

My Evening Wellbeing Markers		Evening Journaling
Hydration ☆☆☆☆☆	Nutrition ☆☆☆☆☆	This is a *Stream of Consciousness Journaling* type of challenge. Simply write down all that comes to your mind below. There is no required outcome here, only to let whatever needs to come out... out. Write for ten minutes and use the blank pages provided at the back if necessary. Just... write!
Daylight/Outside ☆☆☆☆☆	Phone ☆☆☆☆☆	
Total Wellbeing Score		
Tick here when you have completed your habit/action/metric *tracker*.		

Thursday- Date: _____			
My Morning Wellbeing Check-In			**Morning Prompts**
Sleep ☆☆☆☆☆	Energy Levels ☆☆☆☆☆		1. What three things can I do today that will make me feel it was a great day when I reflect before I go to sleep?
Mood ☆☆☆☆☆	Muscle Soreness ☆☆☆☆☆		2. What would it look like for me to live true to my values today?
Total Wellbeing Score			3. Today I want to use the best of my energy to…

_____

Morning Challenge- Rewrite your personal definition of *Success* from memory and then return to page 9 to check for accuracy. Give it your best shot. Don't expect it to be perfect. It doesn't need to be.

_____

My Evening Wellbeing Markers		Evening Prompts
Hydration ☆☆☆☆☆	Nutrition ☆☆☆☆☆	1. What could I have done better today and what are the lessons to be learned from this?
Daylight/Outside ☆☆☆☆☆	Phone ☆☆☆☆☆	2. What is making me proud?
Total Wellbeing Score		3. What intrigues me? What am I curious about?
Tick here when you have completed your habit/action/metric *tracker*.		

Friday- Date: _____			
My Morning Wellbeing Check-In			Morning Prompts
Sleep ☆☆☆☆☆	Energy Levels ☆☆☆☆☆		1. What three things can I do today that will make me feel it was a great day when I reflect before I go to sleep?
Mood ☆☆☆☆☆	Muscle Soreness ☆☆☆☆☆		2. How can I make those around me feel special today?
Total Wellbeing Score			3. I am excited about…

My Evening Wellbeing Markers		Evening Prompts
Hydration ☆☆☆☆☆	Nutrition ☆☆☆☆☆	1. How do you feel you are influencing others in a positive way?
Daylight/Outside ☆☆☆☆☆	Phone ☆☆☆☆☆	2. What did I learn or relearn today?
Total Wellbeing Score		3. For me happiness is to be found...
Tick here when you have completed your habit/action/metric *tracker*.		

Saturday- Date: _____
Time to Reflect and Summarise My Learnings

My Weekly Wellbeing Check-In Averages			
Sleep ☆☆☆☆☆	Energy Levels ☆☆☆☆☆	Hydration ☆☆☆☆☆	Nutrition ☆☆☆☆☆
Mood ☆☆☆☆☆	Muscle Soreness ☆☆☆☆☆	Daylight/Outside ☆☆☆☆☆	Phone ☆☆☆☆☆
My Average Wellness Score			
Out of 5, rate your consistency in using your habit/action/metric tracker			

Based on these scores, I need to:

Start _____

Stop _____

Continue _____

Your challenge is to complete five of these prompts at the very least; maybe more and perhaps even all of them. Simply write the number of the prompt and journal your response in the space provided. This is important work!

1) Note one example of how you lived according to your values/personal mission statement this week and explain how this made you feel.
2) Describe one way your values/personal mission statement were challenged or compromised this week and explain what you learned from this experience.
3) List two things that went well this week inside or outside of sport and offer reasons as to why.
4) What were your two most important learnings or relearnings this week (one inside sport and one outside of sport) and explain how you plan to bring these forward to better yourself?
5) What did you come across this week that you were interested in or were curious about, and would like to look into at a deeper level? How or where can you learn more about this?
6) Think of an example from the past week where you were *fully engaged*. Explain in detail how it felt to be *fully engaged*.
7) What relationships did I improve this week and how?
8) Who helped you this week and how?
9) I was a good teammate this week because…
10) I improved as an athlete this week by…
11) One great moment from the week I want to remember is…
12) My top three accomplishments from the week were:
13) Write a note on the progress you have made this week with regard to achieving your goals.
14) My key takeaways from this week are:

My Four-Week Review

Date: _____

Review your habit/action/metric *tracker* for this four-week block:
1. List the areas where you have shown consistency and progress.
2. List the areas you would like to show more consistency over the next period.

_____
_____
_____
_____
_____
_____
_____

Review your *Wellness Scores* for the past four Saturdays. Based on these scores, I need to:

Start
_____
_____

Stop
_____
_____

Continue
_____
_____

Review your past four weeks journaling, in particular your Saturdays, and …

Select your top two learnings or relearnings from this period.

_____
_____

Select your top two accomplishments from this period.

Select the top two ways you have improved as an athlete over this period.

Select your top two takeaways from this period.

My Next Four Weeks

My Learning Tools

My Learning Tools

My Learning Tools

My Learning Tools

My Goals – My Intentions

Signed: _____ Date: _____

My Goals – My Intentions

Signed: _____ Date: _____

My Tracker

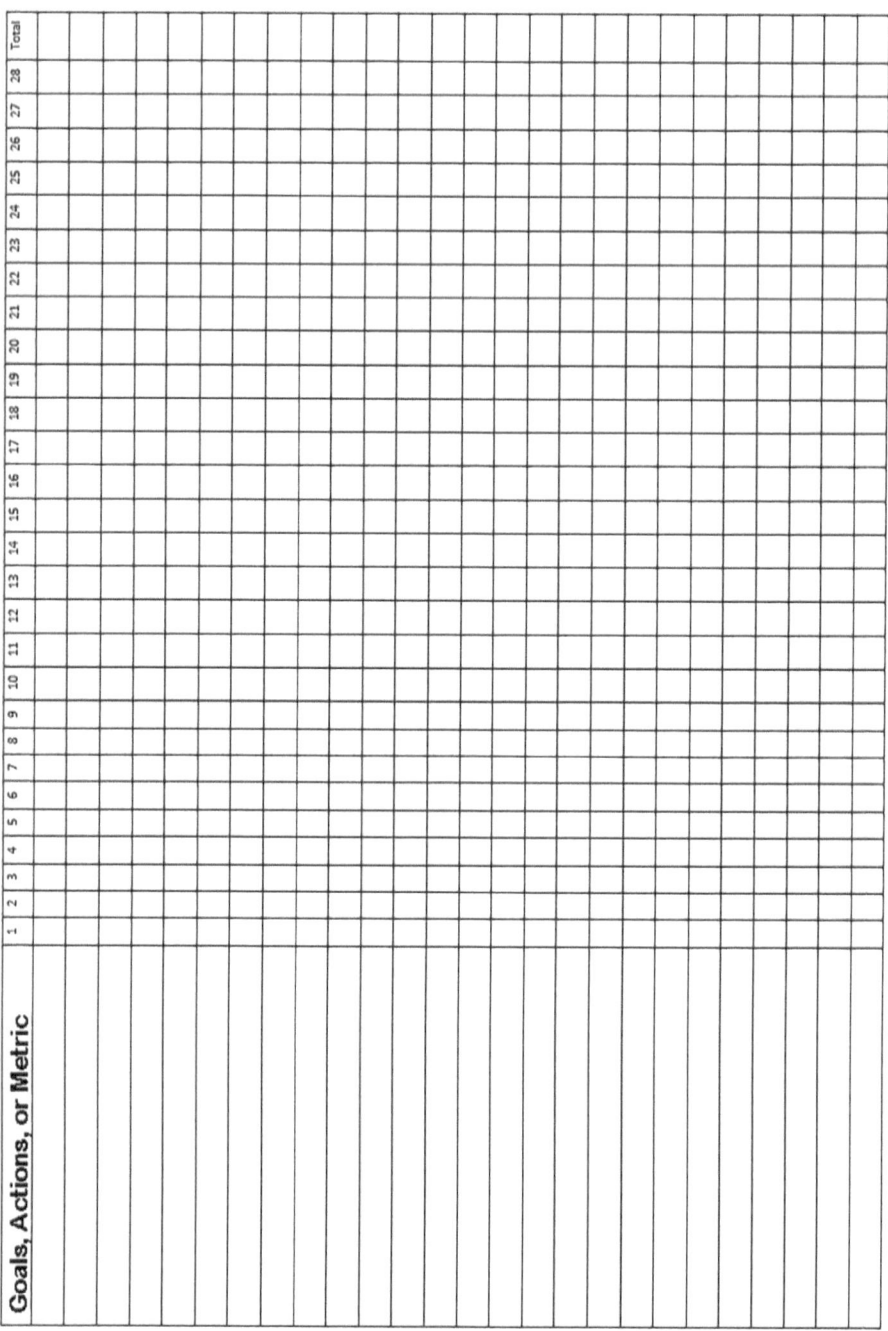

My Next Four Weeks – Important Things

(You can fill in the date in the small boxes provided in the top left-hand corner.)

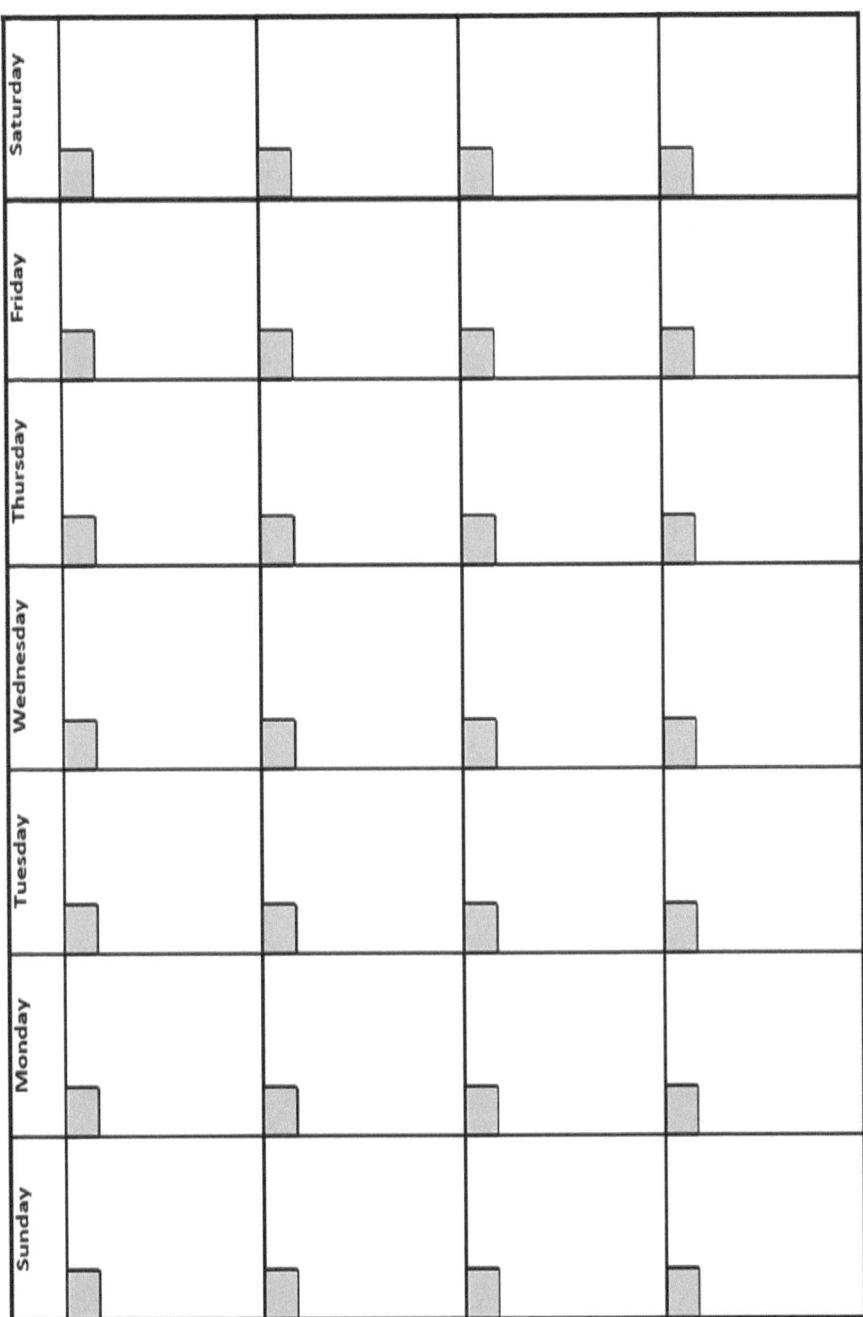

Sunday- Time to Plan for the Week Ahead

Date: _____

Your challenge is to complete three of these prompts at the very least; maybe more and perhaps even all of them. Simply write the number of the prompt and journal your response in the space provided. This is important work!

1) Describe in detail how you intend to live this week. Here you may wish to draw insights from your Values, your *Personal Mission Statement*, and your goals or intentions.
2) List at least one area of your life outside of sport that you would like to live with intention this week and explain the behaviours or actions required to do so.
3) Describe in detail at least one way you are going to improve as a teammate this week and explain how that will make you feel.
4) Describe in detail how you plan to improve as an athlete this week: what tools and practices are you going to utilise, what are your key *work-ons*, who or what can help you, etc.
5) What are the biggest sporting challenges that lay ahead of you this week? How to do want to 'show up' for these?
6) Full engagement is the acquired ability to give your full and best energy and effort to what you are doing at any given moment. Where is the one area you would like to be *fully engaged* this week and why is it important you do so?
7) In order to bring balance, recreation, regeneration and joy to your life this week what hobbies, interests or activities outside of sport do you need to make time for?
8) To help me make progress towards achieving my goals or living my intentions, this week I will...(List five actions.)

Important for the Week Ahead

Here you can use the blank spaces to schedule or craft your plan for the week ahead in whatever format you wish.

Monday	Tuesday	Wednesday

Thursday	Friday	Saturday

Monday- Date: _____			
My Morning Wellbeing Check-In			**Morning Prompts**
Sleep ☆☆☆☆☆	Energy Levels ☆☆☆☆☆		1. What am I grateful for this morning? Explain in detail.
Mood ☆☆☆☆☆	Muscle Soreness ☆☆☆☆☆		2. How do I want to feel today and what am I willing to do to achieve this?
Total Wellbeing Score			3. I will smile when my head hits the pillow this evening if…

_____
_____
_____
_____
_____
_____
_____
_____
_____
_____
_____
_____
_____
_____
_____
_____
_____
_____
_____
_____
_____
_____
_____
_____

Morning Challenge- Return to page 5 and read your *Values* and their definitions three times.

My Evening Wellbeing Markers		Evening Prompts
Hydration ☆☆☆☆☆	Nutrition ☆☆☆☆☆	1. What did I do well today and why/how?
Daylight/Outside ☆☆☆☆☆	Phone ☆☆☆☆☆	2. What did I learn or relearn today?
Total Wellbeing Score		3. What is one thing I could have done better today and how?
Tick here when you have completed your habit/action/metric *tracker*.		

Tuesday- Date: _____

My Morning Wellbeing Check-In		Morning Prompts
Sleep ☆☆☆☆☆	Energy Levels ☆☆☆☆☆	1. What am I grateful for this morning? Explain in detail.
Mood ☆☆☆☆☆	Muscle Soreness ☆☆☆☆☆	2. Who would I like to connect with today and why?
Total Wellbeing Score		3. What can I do in order to inject more fun into the day ahead?

Morning Challenge- Return to page 5 and read your *Values* and their definitions three times.

My Evening Wellbeing Markers		Evening Prompts
Hydration ☆☆☆☆☆	Nutrition ☆☆☆☆☆	1. What were the three best things about today?
Daylight/Outside ☆☆☆☆☆	Phone ☆☆☆☆☆	2. Who did I help today, how did I help them and how did it make me feel? Who could I have helped more?
Total Wellbeing Score		3. Something I am procrastinating over is... What action should I take?
Tick here when you have completed your habit/action/metric *tracker*.		

Wednesday- Date: _____

My Morning Wellbeing Check-In		Morning Prompts
Sleep ☆☆☆☆☆	Energy Levels ☆☆☆☆☆	1. What am I grateful for this morning? Explain in detail.
Mood ☆☆☆☆☆	Muscle Soreness ☆☆☆☆☆	2. Write about a positive experience from yesterday: what was it, why did it come about and how did it make you feel?
Total Wellbeing Score		3. I feel good when I start my day with….

....

Morning Challenge- Rewrite your *Values* and their definitions from memory and then return to page 5 to check for accuracy. Give it your best shot. Don't expect it to be perfect. It doesn't need to be.

....

My Evening Wellbeing Markers		Evening Journaling
Hydration ☆☆☆☆☆	Nutrition ☆☆☆☆☆	This is a *Stream of Consciousness Journaling* type of challenge. Simply write down all that comes to your mind below. There is no required outcome here, only to let whatever needs to come out… out. Write for ten minutes and use the blank pages provided at the back if necessary. Just… write!
Daylight/Outside ☆☆☆☆☆	Phone ☆☆☆☆☆	
Total Wellbeing Score		
Tick here when you have completed your habit/action/metric *tracker*.		

Thursday- Date: _____			
My Morning Wellbeing Check-In			**Morning Prompts**
Sleep ☆☆☆☆☆	Energy Levels ☆☆☆☆☆		1. What am I grateful for this morning? Explain in detail.
Mood ☆☆☆☆☆	Muscle Soreness ☆☆☆☆☆		2. What precisely is adding energy to my life right now?
Total Wellbeing Score			3. What is one thing I can do today to bring more happiness into my day?

Morning Challenge- Read your *Personal Mission Statement* from page 6 three times.

My Evening Wellbeing Markers		Evening Prompts
Hydration ☆☆☆☆☆	Nutrition ☆☆☆☆☆	1. Write about the highlight of your day; think- what, why, when, where, who and how.
Daylight/Outside ☆☆☆☆☆	Phone ☆☆☆☆☆	2. What did I learn or relearn today?
Total Wellbeing Score		3. How did I grow as an athlete and person today?
Tick here when you have completed your habit/action/metric *tracker*.		

Friday- Date: _____

My Morning Wellbeing Check-In		Morning Prompts
Sleep ☆☆☆☆☆	Energy Levels ☆☆☆☆☆	1. What am I grateful for this morning? Explain in detail.
Mood ☆☆☆☆☆	Muscle Soreness ☆☆☆☆☆	2. As I look towards the day ahead write down: two things I can control, two things I can influence and two things I can't control.
Total Wellbeing Score		3 What three things are most important for me today and how can I tend to these?

....
....
....
....
....
....
....
....
....
....
....
....
....
....
....
....

Morning Challenge- Rewrite your *Personal Mission Statement* from memory and then return to page 6 to check for accuracy. Give it your best shot. Don't expect it to be perfect. It doesn't need to be.

....
....
....
....

My Evening Wellbeing Markers		Evening Prompts
Hydration ☆☆☆☆☆	Nutrition ☆☆☆☆☆	1. What is currently bringing the most joy to my life and why?
Daylight/Outside ☆☆☆☆☆	Phone ☆☆☆☆☆	2. My greatest learning resources as an athlete are… (think: who, what, where, how).
Total Wellbeing Score		3. I live true to my values when I…
Tick here when you have completed your habit/action/metric *tracker*.		

Saturday- Date: _____
Time to Reflect and Summarise My Learnings

My Weekly Wellbeing Check-In Averages			
Sleep ☆☆☆☆☆	Energy Levels ☆☆☆☆☆	Hydration ☆☆☆☆☆	Nutrition ☆☆☆☆☆
Mood ☆☆☆☆☆	Muscle Soreness ☆☆☆☆☆	Daylight/Outside ☆☆☆☆☆	Phone ☆☆☆☆☆
My Average Wellness Score			
Out of 5, rate your consistency in using your habit/action/metric tracker			

Based on these scores, I need to:

Start _____

Stop _____

Continue _____

Your challenge is to complete five of these prompts at the very least; maybe more and perhaps even all of them. Simply write the number of the prompt and journal your response in the space provided. This is important work!

1) Note one example of how you lived according to your values/personal mission statement this week and explain how this made you feel.
2) Describe one way your values/personal mission statement were challenged or compromised this week and explain what you learned from this experience.
3) List two things that went well this week inside or outside of sport and offer reasons as to why.
4) What were your two most important learnings or relearnings this week (one inside sport and one outside of sport) and explain how you plan to bring these forward to better yourself?
5) What did you come across this week that you were interested in or were curious about, and would like to look into at a deeper level? How or where can you learn more about this?
6) Think of an example from the past week where you were *fully engaged*. Explain in detail how it felt to be *fully engaged*.
7) What relationships did I improve this week and how?
8) Who helped you this week and how?
9) I was a good teammate this week because…
10) I improved as an athlete this week by…
11) One great moment from the week I want to remember is…
12) My top three accomplishments from the week were:
13) Write a note on the progress you have made this week with regard to achieving your goals.
14) My key takeaways from this week are:

Sunday- Time to Plan for the Week Ahead

Date: _____

Your challenge is to complete three of these prompts at the very least; maybe more and perhaps even all of them. Simply write the number of the prompt and journal your response in the space provided. This is important work!

1) Describe in detail how you intend to live this week. Here you may wish to draw insights from your Values, your *Personal Mission Statement*, and your goals or intentions.
2) List at least one area of your life outside of sport that you would like to live with intention this week and explain the behaviours or actions required to do so.
3) Describe in detail at least one way you are going to improve as a teammate this week and explain how that will make you feel.
4) Describe in detail how you plan to improve as an athlete this week: what tools and practices are you going to utilise, what are your key *work-ons*, who or what can help you, etc.
5) What are the biggest sporting challenges that lay ahead of you this week? How to do want to 'show up' for these?
6) Full engagement is the acquired ability to give your full and best energy and effort to what you are doing at any given moment. Where is the one area you would like to be *fully engaged* this week and why is it important you do so?
7) In order to bring balance, recreation, regeneration and joy to your life this week what hobbies, interests or activities outside of sport do you need to make time for?
8) To help me make progress towards achieving my goals or living my intentions, this week I will...(List five actions.)

Important for the Week Ahead

Here you can use the blank spaces to schedule or craft your plan for the week ahead in whatever format you wish.

Monday	Tuesday	Wednesday
Thursday	Friday	Saturday

Monday- Date: _____			
My Morning Wellbeing Check-In			**Morning Prompts**
Sleep ☆☆☆☆☆	Energy Levels ☆☆☆☆☆		1. List three things that are good about today.
Mood ☆☆☆☆☆	Muscle Soreness ☆☆☆☆☆		2. Write the names of three people you interact with daily. Note at least one positive thing about each of them.
Total Wellbeing Score			3. How can I be kind to myself today?

Morning Challenge- Return to page 6 and read your explanation of, or answer to, 'What Sport Means to Me' three times.

My Evening Wellbeing Markers		Evening Prompts
Hydration ☆☆☆☆☆	Nutrition ☆☆☆☆☆	1. What is currently bringing satisfaction into my life?
Daylight/Outside ☆☆☆☆☆	Phone ☆☆☆☆☆	2. Where in my life am I currently making excuses? How can I improve this?
Total Wellbeing Score		3. I feel good when I end my day with...
Tick here when you have completed your habit/action/metric *tracker*.		

Tuesday- Date: _____			
My Morning Wellbeing Check-In			**Morning Prompts**
Sleep ☆☆☆☆☆		Energy Levels ☆☆☆☆☆	1. List three things that are good about today.
Mood ☆☆☆☆☆		Muscle Soreness ☆☆☆☆☆	2. Who am I when I am at my very best (physically, mentally, spiritually, etc.)? Write between six to ten words that you believe are representative of you when you're most proud of yourself, regardless of circumstance or situation.
Total Wellbeing Score			3. Why is it important to be my authentic self?

....
....
....
....
....
....
....
....
....
....
....

Morning Challenge- Rewrite 'What Sport Means to Me' from memory and then return to page 6 to check for accuracy. Give it your best shot. Don't expect it to be perfect. It doesn't need to be.

....
....
....
....
....

My Evening Wellbeing Markers		Evening Prompts
Hydration ☆☆☆☆☆	Nutrition ☆☆☆☆☆	1. Three ways I was true to my *Values* today:
Daylight/Outside ☆☆☆☆☆	Phone ☆☆☆☆☆	2. List and explain at least two ways you feel like you are influencing others in a positive way.
Total Wellbeing Score		3. I am proud of myself today because…
Tick here when you have completed your habit/action/metric *tracker*.		

Wednesday- Date: _____

My Morning Wellbeing Check-In		Morning Prompts
Sleep ☆☆☆☆☆	Energy Levels ☆☆☆☆☆	1. List three things that are good about today.
Mood ☆☆☆☆☆	Muscle Soreness ☆☆☆☆☆	2. What three things can I do today that will make me feel it was a great day when I reflect before I go to sleep?
Total Wellbeing Score		3. What is my most important 'Value' and why?

Morning Challenge- Return to page 7 and read your explanation for, or answer to, 'My Vision for Myself as a Teammate' three times.

My Evening Wellbeing Markers		Evening Journaling
Hydration ☆☆☆☆☆	Nutrition ☆☆☆☆☆	This is a *Stream of Consciousness Journaling* type of challenge. Simply write down all that comes to your mind below. There is no required outcome here, only to let whatever needs to come out... out. Write for ten minutes and use the blank pages provided at the back if necessary. Just... write!
Daylight/Outside ☆☆☆☆☆	Phone ☆☆☆☆☆	
Total Wellbeing Score		
Tick here when you have completed your habit/action/metric *tracker*.		

Thursday- Date: _____	
My Morning Wellbeing Check-In		**Morning Prompts**
Sleep ☆☆☆☆☆	Energy Levels ☆☆☆☆☆	1. List three things that are good about today.
Mood ☆☆☆☆☆	Muscle Soreness ☆☆☆☆☆	2. Write up a rough plan for the day ahead. Include the major events in your day and note how you wish to turn up and present yourself in each of these situations.
Total Wellbeing Score		3. Today I will...

Morning Challenge- Rewrite your 'My Vision for Myself as a Teammate' from memory and then return to page 7 to check for accuracy. Give it your best shot. Don't expect it to be perfect. It doesn't need to be.

My Evening Wellbeing Markers		Evening Prompts
Hydration ☆☆☆☆☆	Nutrition ☆☆☆☆☆	1. List three things that were good about today.
Daylight/Outside ☆☆☆☆☆	Phone ☆☆☆☆☆	2. Describe your biggest learning or relearning from today.
Total Wellbeing Score		3. Who helped me today and how did they help me?
Tick here when you have completed your habit/action/metric *tracker*.		

Friday- Date: _____

My Morning Wellbeing Check-In		Morning Prompts
Sleep ☆☆☆☆☆	Energy Levels ☆☆☆☆☆	1. List three things that are good about today.
Mood ☆☆☆☆☆	Muscle Soreness ☆☆☆☆☆	2. How/Where/To whom do I want to show kindness today?
Total Wellbeing Score		3 What three things are most important to me for the day ahead?

My Evening Wellbeing Markers		Evening Prompts
Hydration ☆ ☆ ☆ ☆ ☆	Nutrition ☆ ☆ ☆ ☆ ☆	1. What did I do well today and why/how?
Daylight/Outside ☆ ☆ ☆ ☆ ☆	Phone ☆ ☆ ☆ ☆ ☆	2. Return to this morning's journal prompt where you were asked to list three things you felt were most important for you for the day ahead. Did you tend to these things in a satisfactory manner? If the answer is Yes: explain how this makes you feel. If the answer is No: explain your strongest reason for not doing it.
Total Wellbeing Score		3. What are the habits, behaviours or distractions that pull me away from being present or in the moment?
Tick here when you have completed your habit/action/metric *tracker*.		

Saturday- Date: _____
Time to Reflect and Summarise My Learnings

My Weekly Wellbeing Check-In Averages			
Sleep ☆☆☆☆☆	Energy Levels ☆☆☆☆☆	Hydration ☆☆☆☆☆	Nutrition ☆☆☆☆☆
Mood ☆☆☆☆☆	Muscle Soreness ☆☆☆☆☆	Daylight/Outside ☆☆☆☆☆	Phone ☆☆☆☆☆
My Average Wellness Score			
Out of 5, rate your consistency in using your habit/action/metric tracker			

Based on these scores, I need to:

Start ....

Stop ....

Continue ....

Your challenge is to complete five of these prompts at the very least; maybe more and perhaps even all of them. Simply write the number of the prompt and journal your response in the space provided. This is important work!

1) Note one example of how you lived according to your values/personal mission statement this week and explain how this made you feel.
2) Describe one way your values/personal mission statement were challenged or compromised this week and explain what you learned from this experience.
3) List two things that went well this week inside or outside of sport and offer reasons as to why.
4) What were your two most important learnings or relearnings this week (one inside sport and one outside of sport) and explain how you plan to bring these forward to better yourself?
5) What did you come across this week that you were interested in or were curious about, and would like to look into at a deeper level? How or where can you learn more about this?
6) Think of an example from the past week where you were *fully engaged*. Explain in detail how it felt to be *fully engaged*.
7) What relationships did I improve this week and how?
8) Who helped you this week and how?
9) I was a good teammate this week because...
10) I improved as an athlete this week by...
11) One great moment from the week I want to remember is...
12) My top three accomplishments from the week were:
13) Write a note on the progress you have made this week with regard to achieving your goals.
14) My key takeaways from this week are:

Sunday- Time to Plan for the Week Ahead

Date: _____

Your challenge is to complete three of these prompts at the very least; maybe more and perhaps even all of them. Simply write the number of the prompt and journal your response in the space provided. This is important work!

1) Describe in detail how you intend to live this week. Here you may wish to draw insights from your Values, your *Personal Mission Statement*, and your goals or intentions.
2) List at least one area of your life outside of sport that you would like to live with intention this week and explain the behaviours or actions required to do so.
3) Describe in detail at least one way you are going to improve as a teammate this week and explain how that will make you feel.
4) Describe in detail how you plan to improve as an athlete this week: what tools and practices are you going to utilise, what are your key *work-ons*, who or what can help you, etc.
5) What are the biggest sporting challenges that lay ahead of you this week? How to do want to 'show up' for these?
6) Full engagement is the acquired ability to give your full and best energy and effort to what you are doing at any given moment. Where is the one area you would like to be *fully engaged* this week and why is it important you do so?
7) In order to bring balance, recreation, regeneration and joy to your life this week what hobbies, interests or activities outside of sport do you need to make time for?
8) To help me make progress towards achieving my goals or living my intentions, this week I will…(List five actions.)

Important for the Week Ahead

Here you can use the blank spaces to schedule or craft your plan for the week ahead in whatever format you wish.

Monday	Tuesday	Wednesday

Thursday	Friday	Saturday

Monday- Date: _____			
My Morning Wellbeing Check-In			**Morning Prompts**
Sleep ☆☆☆☆☆		Energy Levels ☆☆☆☆☆	1. Complete this sentence three times: I am grateful for ... because...
Mood ☆☆☆☆☆		Muscle Soreness ☆☆☆☆☆	2. Name one area you would like to be *fully engaged* today and explain why. We will refer to it this evening as your *fully engaged target area*.
Total Wellbeing Score			3. Write down some core principles for the day- What principles do I want to live by today?

_____
_____
_____
_____
_____
_____
_____
_____
_____
_____
_____
_____
_____
_____
_____
_____
_____
_____
_____
_____

Morning Challenge- Return to page 8 and read your explanation of, or answer to, 'My truth or belief around application to collective and individual practice' three times

My Evening Wellbeing Markers		Evening Prompts
Hydration ☆☆☆☆☆	Nutrition ☆☆☆☆☆	1. How did your *fully engaged target area* from this morning play out for you? What lessons did you learn?
Daylight/Outside ☆☆☆☆☆	Phone ☆☆☆☆☆	2. Where have I been doing well of late? In what areas have I been growing?
Total Wellbeing Score		3. What am I currently finding inspiring?
Tick here when you have completed your habit/action/metric *tracker*.		

Tuesday- Date: _____

My Morning Wellbeing Check-In		Morning Prompts
Sleep ☆☆☆☆☆	Energy Levels ☆☆☆☆☆	1. Complete this sentence three times: I am grateful for ... because...
Mood ☆☆☆☆☆	Muscle Soreness ☆☆☆☆☆	2. Describe how you can behave and prepare like a champion today.
Total Wellbeing Score		3. Finish the following- I am... I can... I will...

Morning Challenge- Rewrite your 'My truth or belief around application to collective and individual practice' from memory and then return to page 8 to check for accuracy. Give it your best shot. Don't expect it to be perfect. It doesn't need to be.

My Evening Wellbeing Markers		Evening Prompts
Hydration ☆☆☆☆☆	Nutrition ☆☆☆☆☆	1. Champions consistently make good choices. Make a list of 'champion choices'.
Daylight/Outside ☆☆☆☆☆	Phone ☆☆☆☆☆	2. What did I learn or relearn today?
Total Wellbeing Score		3. Write about an area in your life where you feel stuck right now and how you can begin to make progress here.
Tick here when you have completed your habit/action/metric *tracker*.		

Wednesday- Date: _____		
My Morning Wellbeing Check-In		**Morning Prompts**
Sleep ☆☆☆☆☆	Energy Levels ☆☆☆☆☆	1. Complete this sentence three times: I am grateful for ... because...
Mood ☆☆☆☆☆	Muscle Soreness ☆☆☆☆☆	2. How can I have a positive impact on others today?
Total Wellbeing Score		3. Today I will nourish my body and mind by...

Morning Challenge- Return to page 9 and read your personal definition of *Excellence* three times.

My Evening Wellbeing Markers		Evening Journaling
Hydration ☆☆☆☆☆	Nutrition ☆☆☆☆☆	This is a *Stream of Consciousness Journaling* type of challenge. Simply write down all that comes to your mind below. There is no required outcome here, only to let whatever needs to come out... out. Write for ten minutes and use the blank pages provided at the back if necessary. Just... write!
Daylight/Outside ☆☆☆☆☆	Phone ☆☆☆☆☆	
Total Wellbeing Score		
Tick here when you have completed your habit/action/metric *tracker*.		

Thursday- Date: _____			
My Morning Wellbeing Check-In			**Morning Prompts**
Sleep ☆☆☆☆☆	Energy Levels ☆☆☆☆☆		1. Complete this sentence three times: I am grateful for ... because...
Mood ☆☆☆☆☆	Muscle Soreness ☆☆☆☆☆		2. Write for five minutes... 'I feel happiest when...' let it flow.
Total Wellbeing Score			3. How do I plan to grow as an athlete and person today?

Morning Challenge- Rewrite your personal definition of *Excellence* from memory and then return to page 9 to check for accuracy. Give it your best shot. Don't expect it to be perfect. It doesn't need to be.

My Evening Wellbeing Markers		Evening Prompts
Hydration ☆☆☆☆☆	Nutrition ☆☆☆☆☆	1. Much of sport involves dealing with discomfort, challenge and pressure. Write out a clear vision of how you want to show up in times of discomfort, challenge, and pressure. Take your time here; go deep, bring clarity.
Daylight/Outside ☆☆☆☆☆	Phone ☆☆☆☆☆	2. Where am I making real progress and why?
Total Wellbeing Score		3. I can add more depth to my life by…
Tick here when you have completed your habit/action/metric *tracker*.		

Friday- Date: _____

My Morning Wellbeing Check-In		Morning Prompts
Sleep ☆☆☆☆☆	Energy Levels ☆☆☆☆☆	1. Complete this sentence three times: I am grateful for ... because...
Mood ☆☆☆☆☆	Muscle Soreness ☆☆☆☆☆	2. Explain how you can bring your values into your interactions and experiences today.
Total Wellbeing Score		3. I find meaning and purpose in...

My Evening Wellbeing Markers		Evening Prompts
Hydration ☆☆☆☆☆	Nutrition ☆☆☆☆☆	1. What do I need to do more of and why?
Daylight/Outside ☆☆☆☆☆	Phone ☆☆☆☆☆	2. What do I need to do less of and why?
Total Wellbeing Score		3. What do I need to keep doing and why?
Tick here when you have completed your habit/action/metric *tracker*.		

Saturday- Date: _____

Time to Reflect and Summarise My Learnings

My Weekly Wellbeing Check-In Averages			
Sleep ☆☆☆☆☆	Energy Levels ☆☆☆☆☆	Hydration ☆☆☆☆☆	Nutrition ☆☆☆☆☆
Mood ☆☆☆☆☆	Muscle Soreness ☆☆☆☆☆	Daylight/Outside ☆☆☆☆☆	Phone ☆☆☆☆☆
My Average Wellness Score			
Out of 5, rate your consistency in using your habit/action/metric tracker			

Based on these scores, I need to:

Start _____

Stop _____

Continue _____

Your challenge is to complete five of these prompts at the very least; maybe more and perhaps even all of them. Simply write the number of the prompt and journal your response in the space provided. This is important work!

1) Note one example of how you lived according to your values/personal mission statement this week and explain how this made you feel.
2) Describe one way your values/personal mission statement were challenged or compromised this week and explain what you learned from this experience.
3) List two things that went well this week inside or outside of sport and offer reasons as to why.
4) What were your two most important learnings or relearnings this week (one inside sport and one outside of sport) and explain how you plan to bring these forward to better yourself?
5) What did you come across this week that you were interested in or were curious about, and would like to look into at a deeper level? How or where can you learn more about this?
6) Think of an example from the past week where you were *fully engaged*. Explain in detail how it felt to be *fully engaged*.
7) What relationships did I improve this week and how?
8) Who helped you this week and how?
9) I was a good teammate this week because…
10) I improved as an athlete this week by…
11) One great moment from the week I want to remember is…
12) My top three accomplishments from the week were:
13) Write a note on the progress you have made this week with regard to achieving your goals.
14) My key takeaways from this week are:

Sunday- Time to Plan for the Week Ahead

Date: _____

Your challenge is to complete three of these prompts at the very least; maybe more and perhaps even all of them. Simply write the number of the prompt and journal your response in the space provided. This is important work!

1) Describe in detail how you intend to live this week. Here you may wish to draw insights from your Values, your *Personal Mission Statement*, and your goals or intentions.
2) List at least one area of your life outside of sport that you would like to live with intention this week and explain the behaviours or actions required to do so.
3) Describe in detail at least one way you are going to improve as a teammate this week and explain how that will make you feel.
4) Describe in detail how you plan to improve as an athlete this week: what tools and practices are you going to utilise, what are your key *work-ons*, who or what can help you, etc.
5) What are the biggest sporting challenges that lay ahead of you this week? How to do want to 'show up' for these?
6) Full engagement is the acquired ability to give your full and best energy and effort to what you are doing at any given moment. Where is the one area you would like to be *fully engaged* this week and why is it important you do so?
7) In order to bring balance, recreation, regeneration and joy to your life this week what hobbies, interests or activities outside of sport do you need to make time for?
8) To help me make progress towards achieving my goals or living my intentions, this week I will…(List five actions.)

Important for the Week Ahead

Here you can use the blank spaces to schedule or craft your plan for the week ahead in whatever format you wish.

Monday	Tuesday	Wednesday

Thursday	Friday	Saturday

Monday- Date: _____			
My Morning Wellbeing Check-In			**Morning Prompts**
Sleep ☆☆☆☆☆	Energy Levels ☆☆☆☆☆		1. What three things can I do today that will make me feel it was a great day when I reflect before I go to sleep?
Mood ☆☆☆☆☆	Muscle Soreness ☆☆☆☆☆		2. What relationships would I like to strengthen today and how can I do this?
Total Wellbeing Score			3. Something I've been putting off that I can do today is…

_____

Morning Challenge- Return to page 9 and read your personal definition of *Commitment* three times.

My Evening Wellbeing Markers		Evening Prompts
Hydration ☆☆☆☆☆	Nutrition ☆☆☆☆☆	1. What did I do well today and why/how?
Daylight/Outside ☆☆☆☆☆	Phone ☆☆☆☆☆	2. What is currently bringing energy to my life?
Total Wellbeing Score		3. What is currently draining me and what can I do to overcome this?
Tick here when you have completed your habit/action/metric *tracker*.		

Tuesday- Date: _____

My Morning Wellbeing Check-In		Morning Prompts
Sleep ☆☆☆☆☆	Energy Levels ☆☆☆☆☆	1. What three things can I do today that will make me feel it was a great day when I reflect before I go to sleep?
Mood ☆☆☆☆☆	Muscle Soreness ☆☆☆☆☆	2. How can I add more fun to my day today?
Total Wellbeing Score		3. List three benefits of journaling, planning and tracking.

_____
_____
_____
_____
_____
_____
_____
_____
_____
_____
_____
_____
_____

Morning Challenge- Rewrite your personal definition of *Commitment* from memory and then return to page 9 to check for accuracy. Give it your best shot. Don't expect it to be perfect. It doesn't need to be.

_____
_____
_____
_____

My Evening Wellbeing Markers		Evening Prompts
Hydration ☆☆☆☆☆	Nutrition ☆☆☆☆☆	1. Write about one great moment from today in detail.
Daylight/Outside ☆☆☆☆☆	Phone ☆☆☆☆☆	2. In general, what is something that makes you feel knocked off course, reactive, and not at your personal best? Why do you feel this is so?
Total Wellbeing Score		3. It's hard for me to open up about...
Tick here when you have completed your habit/action/metric *tracker*.		

Wednesday- Date: _____			
My Morning Wellbeing Check-In			**Morning Prompts**
Sleep ☆☆☆☆☆	Energy Levels ☆☆☆☆☆		1. What three things can I do today that will make me feel it was a great day when I reflect before I go to sleep?
Mood ☆☆☆☆☆	Muscle Soreness ☆☆☆☆☆		2. What can I do today to make me feel more connected to other people?
Total Wellbeing Score			3. I would feel lighter if I let go of…

Morning Challenge- Return to page 9 and read your personal definition of *Success* three times.

My Evening Wellbeing Markers		Evening Journaling
Hydration ☆☆☆☆☆	Nutrition ☆☆☆☆☆	This is a *Stream of Consciousness Journaling* type of challenge. Simply write down all that comes to your mind below. There is no required outcome here, only to let whatever needs to come out... out. Write for ten minutes and use the blank pages provided at the back if necessary. Just... write!
Daylight/Outside ☆☆☆☆☆	Phone ☆☆☆☆☆	
Total Wellbeing Score		
Tick here when you have completed your habit/action/metric *tracker*.		

Thursday- Date: _____			
My Morning Wellbeing Check-In		**Morning Prompts**	
Sleep ☆☆☆☆☆	Energy Levels ☆☆☆☆☆	1. What three things can I do today that will make me feel it was a great day when I reflect before I go to sleep?	
Mood ☆☆☆☆☆	Muscle Soreness ☆☆☆☆☆	2. What would it look like for me to live true to my values today?	
Total Wellbeing Score		3. Today I want to use the best of my energy to…	

Morning Challenge- Rewrite your personal definition of *Success* from memory and then return to page 9 to check for accuracy. Give it your best shot. Don't expect it to be perfect. It doesn't need to be.

My Evening Wellbeing Markers		Evening Prompts
Hydration ☆☆☆☆☆	Nutrition ☆☆☆☆☆	1. What could I have done better today and what are the lessons to be learned from this?
Daylight/Outside ☆☆☆☆☆	Phone ☆☆☆☆☆	2. What is making me proud?
Total Wellbeing Score		3. What intrigues me? What am I curious about?
Tick here when you have completed your habit/action/metric *tracker*.		

Friday- Date: _____

My Morning Wellbeing Check-In		Morning Prompts
Sleep ☆☆☆☆☆	Energy Levels ☆☆☆☆☆	1. What three things can I do today that will make me feel it was a great day when I reflect before I go to sleep?
Mood ☆☆☆☆☆	Muscle Soreness ☆☆☆☆☆	2. How can I make those around me feel special today?
Total Wellbeing Score		3. I am excited about…

My Evening Wellbeing Markers		Evening Prompts
Hydration ☆☆☆☆☆	Nutrition ☆☆☆☆☆	1. How do you feel you are influencing others in a positive way?
Daylight/Outside ☆☆☆☆☆	Phone ☆☆☆☆☆	2. What did I learn or relearn today?
Total Wellbeing Score		3. For me happiness is to be found…
Tick here when you have completed your habit/action/metric *tracker*.		

Saturday- Date: _____
Time to Reflect and Summarise My Learnings

My Weekly Wellbeing Check-In Averages			
Sleep ☆☆☆☆☆	Energy Levels ☆☆☆☆☆	Hydration ☆☆☆☆☆	Nutrition ☆☆☆☆☆
Mood ☆☆☆☆☆	Muscle Soreness ☆☆☆☆☆	Daylight/Outside ☆☆☆☆☆	Phone ☆☆☆☆☆
My Average Wellness Score			
Out of 5, rate your consistency in using your habit/action/metric tracker			

Based on these scores, I need to:

Start ....

Stop ....

Continue ....

Your challenge is to complete five of these prompts at the very least; maybe more and perhaps even all of them. Simply write the number of the prompt and journal your response in the space provided. This is important work!

1) Note one example of how you lived according to your values/personal mission statement this week and explain how this made you feel.
2) Describe one way your values/personal mission statement were challenged or compromised this week and explain what you learned from this experience.
3) List two things that went well this week inside or outside of sport and offer reasons as to why.
4) What were your two most important learnings or relearnings this week (one inside sport and one outside of sport) and explain how you plan to bring these forward to better yourself?
5) What did you come across this week that you were interested in or were curious about, and would like to look into at a deeper level? How or where can you learn more about this?
6) Think of an example from the past week where you were *fully engaged*. Explain in detail how it felt to be *fully engaged*.
7) What relationships did I improve this week and how?
8) Who helped you this week and how?
9) I was a good teammate this week because…
10) I improved as an athlete this week by…
11) One great moment from the week I want to remember is…
12) My top three accomplishments from the week were:
13) Write a note on the progress you have made this week with regard to achieving your goals.
14) My key takeaways from this week are:

My Four-Week Review

Date: _____

Review your habit/action/metric *tracker* for this four-week block:
1. List the areas where you have shown consistency and progress.
2. List the areas you would like to show more consistency over the next period.

_____
_____
_____
_____
_____
_____
_____

Review your *Wellness Scores* for the past four Saturdays. Based on these scores, I need to:

Start
_____

Stop
_____

Continue
_____

Review your past four weeks journaling, in particular your Saturdays, and …

Select your top two learnings or relearnings from this period.

_____
_____

Select your top two accomplishments from this period.

Select the top two ways you have improved as an athlete over this period.

Select your top two takeaways from this period.

My Quarterly Review

My Quarterly Review

Date: _____

Review the three, four-week reviews you have completed this quarter (see pages 96, 180, and 264) and complete the following questions:

List the areas where you have shown consistency and progress throughout this quarter.

....

....

....

....

....

....

List the areas you would like to show more consistency in the next quarter.

....

....

....

....

....

....

What are the big takeaways from your *Wellnes Scores* over this quarter? Consider this in depth. What is the data you have collected telling you?

....

....

....

....

....

....

Select your top three learnings or relearnings from this quarter.

Select your top three accomplishments from this quarter.

Select the top three ways you have improved as an athlete over this quarter.

Select your top three takeaways from this quarter.

What have you learned from completing this quarterly review exercise?

My New 'This is Me' Guide

The beginning of this quarterly journal challenged you to reflect on your learnings to date and harvest them into a cohesive and usable 'Personal Manifesto' or 'This is Me' guide. Since completing this guide 12 weeks ago, you will have reflected further on many of these topics and will hopefully have gained much new insight and perspective.

Below, I have provided the same list of questions; in many ways, we are going back to the start once more. Although we are nearing the end of this journal, I have learned that in life, the end is always the beginning. Being the best you can be in sport requires a relentless pursuit of learning, adapting, refining and improving.

Your challenge here is to rewrite, amend, or adapt as you please. You should use your 'This is Me' guide from the beginning of this quarter as a reference or starting point. You may wish to change a little; you may wish to change a lot. It is totally up to you in how you approach this.

This is Me

My name is _____

I am more than just a _____
(Sport you play)

I play _____

The areas of my life that are most important to me are:
_____
_____
_____
_____
_____

My *Values* are: (Please add a definition or standard of behaviour for each one.)
_____
_____
_____
_____
_____
_____
_____
_____
_____
_____
_____
_____
_____
_____
_____

This is Me

My *Personal Mission Statement* is:

_____
_____
_____
_____
_____
_____
_____

What sport means to me:

_____
_____
_____
_____
_____
_____
_____

I want to be remembered by those I played sport with and against as someone who:

_____
_____
_____
_____
_____
_____
_____

This is Me

My vision for myself as a teammate is:

___
___
___
___
___
___
___

As an athlete, my current *weapons* are:

___
___
___
___

As an athlete, my current *work-ons* are:

___
___
___
___

To ensure I learn as I go in sport, I utilise the following tools and practices:

___
___
___
___
___
___
___

This is Me

My truth or belief around application to collective and individual practice is: (i.e. how I believe one should best apply themselves to practice.)

_____
_____
_____
_____
_____
_____

The activities and hobbies outside of sport that give me energy, bring me joy and add balance to my life are:

_____
_____
_____
_____
_____
_____

With regard to how I spend my time and energy, I aim to be a person who:

_____
_____
_____
_____
_____
_____
_____

This is Me

My personal definition of *Excellence* is:
_____
_____
_____
_____
_____

My personal definition of *Commitment* is:
_____
_____
_____
_____
_____

My personal definition of *Success* is:
_____
_____
_____
_____
_____

Anything else you'd like to add:
_____
_____
_____

Signed: _____ **Date:** _____

Reflections on 12 Weeks of Journaling

Describe how you have enjoyed your past 12 weeks of journaling.

Explain how you feel it has helped and improved you as a person.

Explain how you feel it has helped and improved you as an athlete.

Explain what you see as the advantages of continuing journaling and embedding it as a habit as you moved forward.

The End is Always the Beginning

Congratulations on completing this quarterly journal. It is a super achievement and one you should be proud of. I hope this journal has been of genuine service to you and that you have enjoyed and benefited from the time and energy you have invested in the process.

One of life's great truisms is that the end is always the beginning, and so I hope that you are ready to continue your journaling journey. Consistency is key in journaling. Life and sport continues to challenge us every single day of our lives, and so we must continue the practices that enable us to meet these challenges with strength, clarity and conviction.

You can continue your journaling any way you please. To support your efforts and to sustain this excellent practice, I have carefully crafted this journal as a tool that can be used long-term in a cyclical manner…one after another. If you are wondering how to proceed in your journaling, I suggest that when the time is right for you, begin a new quarterly journal where you left off with this one. Your new 'This is Me' guide, which you have just completed, will act as a starting point. The process of learning and improvement will continue as you continue to pursue the practice of journaling for wellbeing and improved sporting performance.

Be the best you can be,

Paul Kilgannon

P.S. You can purchase your next journal directly from my website www.carvercoachingframework.com or wherever you purchased this one.

www.ingramcontent.com/pod-product-compliance
Lightning Source LLC
Chambersburg PA
CBHW022041160426
43209CB00002B/32

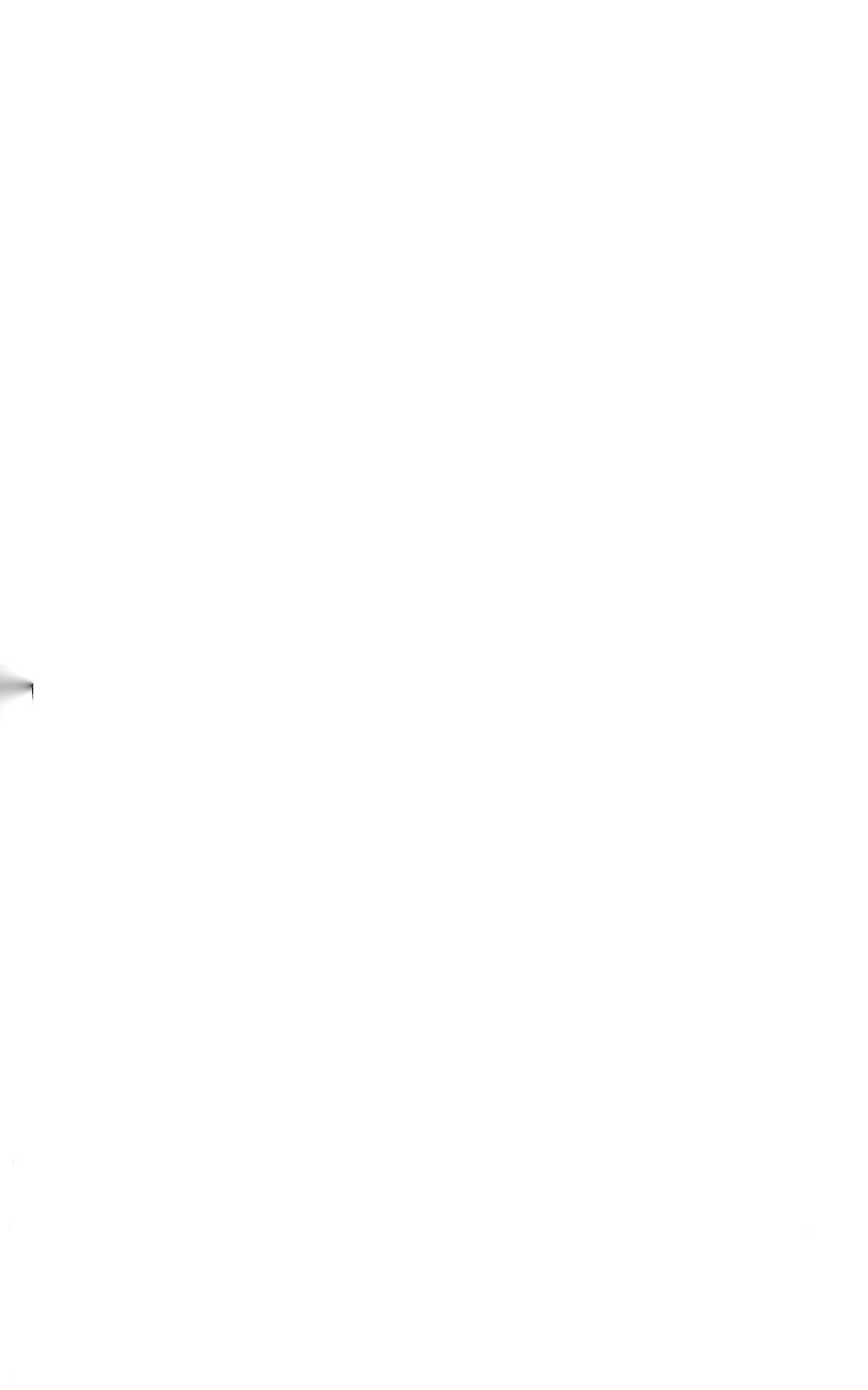